DR TONY REDMOND OBE wa
years and is Emeritus Professo
Medicine at the University of M
NGO UK-Med, he has also worked with the UN, DFID, and the
WHO to deliver emergency care to those most in need around the
world. He has, in the course of his work, been subjected to heavy
metal poisoning, survived malaria and broken his back.

DR JOHN ... has an A&E doctor for over thirty years ... and a senior lecturer of International Emergency Medicine at ... Manchester, UK. Founder of the ...

DR TONY REDMOND

FRONT LINE

STORIES OF CARE AND COURAGE IN EMERGENCY MEDICINE

Harper
North

HarperNorth
Windmill Green,
Mount Street,
Manchester, M2 3NX

A division of
HarperCollins*Publishers*
1 London Bridge Street
London SE1 9GF

www.harpercollins.co.uk

HarperCollins*Publishers*
1st Floor, Watermarque Building, Ringsend Road
Dublin 4, Ireland

First published by HarperNorth in 2021
This revised and updated paperback edition published 2022

1 3 5 7 9 10 8 6 4 2

A catalogue record for this book
is available from the British Library

HB ISBN: 978-0-00-844953-7
PB ISBN: 978-0-00-844956-8

Printed and bound in the UK using 100%
renewable electricity at CPI Group (UK) Ltd

To my family, who have supported me
through good times and bad.

Contents

Foreword

I feel very privileged to have been invited to contribute this fore-word to Tony Redmond's moving and inspiring book.

He is above all a humanitarian, whose calling as a doctor has taken him all over the world. He has faced danger, battled bureau-cracy, made do with very little and overcome obstacles that would have thwarted less determined people. From his close-knit upbring-ing and decision to study medicine, he has given long service to the NHS and to countless people who probably never knew his name but who found themselves in his capable care amid war, famine and disease. Dr Redmond is a man who has clearly done more, much more, than his bit.

This is, however, not just a tale of one person's heroic achievements, although many examples of heroism are to be found here. What is so engaging about this book is that Tony Redmond is searingly honest about the choices he has made and the impact they have had upon him, his family, his colleagues and his health – although I suspect he would never have had it any other way. Throughout, he has striven to adhere to the humanitarian principles of humanity, neutrality, impartiality and independence and to apply them by that most basic step – turning up to help.

He is honest about the fear that he felt and the ambiguities and compromises he has had to confront in trying to assist. From the horror of Lockerbie to the bitter ethnic conflict of Sarajevo and from the ebola outbreak to the earthquake in Haiti, time and time again he had to ask himself 'who should I help?' It is the dilemma that every humanitarian encounters, and he sums up his approach with these wise words: 'I have always worked on the basis that just because I can't do everything for everyone, that must not mean that I can't do something for someone.' I wholeheartedly agree. Life will disappoint if we think it is about seeking perfection. It is mostly about doing what we can when we can, and that Tony Redmond has done in abundance.

There is a contemporary feel to this book as Redmond draws on the parallels between his role in setting up the Manchester Nightingale hospital to treat Covid patients and the work he has done in many countries, and he spares nothing in his criticism of the UK's lack of preparation for the pandemic and of the current Government's decision to abolish DFID and cut our aid budget.

We also meet a range of people that Dr Redmond has worked with who showed great courage, like the nurse who called on him one night for a second opinion on a patient because she didn't trust the judgement of the doctor: she was right. We hear tales of kindness that will make you weep and tales of horror that will make you wonder what happened to common humanity. But of cynicism, Dr Redmond rightly observes: 'cynicism produces nothing and looks to justify doing nothing.'

The other thing this book does is to encourage us to reflect on the effectiveness of the international humanitarian system.

Foreword

Although it has improved quite a bit over the years, it is still not fully functioning. We do not have an international crisis service and the truth remains that the bulk of the care is provided by the country where the disaster takes place. He is very frank about the impact that politics, media coverage and institutional rivalry can have on responding to a crisis, both for good and ill, and he observes that what people often feel is the best thing to do to help does not always end up being useful. Money – rather than donations in kind – is a much more effective means of providing practical assistance, because it can be used to procure exactly what is needed.

Reflecting on his life's experiences at the end of this wonderful book, Dr Redmond writes of the 'desire to do good, to lead a worthy life.' I only hope he knows that his life has been worthy beyond measure.

The Right Honourable Hilary Benn MP
Former Shadow Foreign Secretary
Former Secretary of State for International Development

Timeline

Preface

I am the youngest son, and the next to youngest child, of six offspring born to Liverpool Irish catholic parents, transplanted by the fickleness of love and war to the small Methodist Lancashire mill town of Failsworth. I was born in Manchester itself, in Beech Mount maternity home.

From the grinding poverty of his Everton home, my father had sailed as a young man to South America to train as a priest in a contemplative order. On dark winter nights he would tell me tales of gauchos creeping on their haunches in the stillness of the pampas at night to silently listen outside the mud huts of isolated haciendas. When they heard the steady breathing of sleep, they would slide their long knives through the soft mud wall and into their unknowing victim. If ever I were to find myself travelling alone on the pampas, he told me, I could kill a sheep and eat it. There were so many it was no crime. However, I must first skin the sheep and leave the fleece over a fence. It was valuable; taking it would be stealing.

My knowledge of what to do when travelling alone on the Argentine pampas fortified me for the rigours of life growing up on the edge of Manchester in the 1950s and 60s. My father could bring the smell of oxen roasting over an open fire into the ice-cold winter of our small house, where we sat huddled around the only fire. The house had no central heating; baths were limited to once a week, and even then we often had to share the water. Being at the younger end of a large family is no fun when the order of entry into the rapidly cooling and increasingly grimy bath water is determined by age, I can tell you.

My father hated the English winters. His job involved mostly outdoor industrial work. To survive he took himself off and back to his youth in the sun and space of the Argentine. If I was patient, and lucky, I could catch him in a mood where I could tease this out from his memory and into the world around me. I asked him once why he left the religious order and did not proceed to being a priest? He surprised me by saying that it was too easy; too soft. He had joined to give of himself, to make a sacrifice for the good of others, and all he did was get fat, for the one and only time in his life. When he told the Abbot, he was put in a monk's cell to think over his decision, alone and in silence. When dawn came and he confirmed that he was still of the same mind, he was given back the battered small suitcase he had hauled from home, removed his monk's habit, and re-dressed in his secular clothes. It was when he had difficulty fastening his trousers and the belt had to be let out several notches that he knew he had made the right decision.

He had been brought up in poverty, one of nine children, with sacking nailed over the windows where glass should be, his itinerant father somewhere overseas, and the family just surviving: his mother taking in both washing and lodgers. He told me with such deep conviction how those who talked of the nobility of poverty can never have experienced it for themselves. There was nothing noble about poverty; it was degrading, wearing, and dehumanising. The monks were playing at poverty he said, when he'd known the real thing. All my experience of humanitarian emergencies shows me the same; that at the root of a person's, a country's vulnerability, lies their poverty. A poverty that imprisons them and robs them of even basic chances, including the chance to live. And people do not wish to be poor. They may equally not wish to be rich, but they never wish to be poor. People are kept in poverty by those of us who ignore or profit from their plight.

My father worked all his life to provide for his large family and took little if anything for himself. He never owned a car or opened a bank account. He had one pair of shoes at a time, splattered like a Jackson Pollock from his work, but painted black when the priest visited. He was buried in his only suit – bought at great expense six months earlier – for my graduation as a doctor.

My mother was working for Littlewoods Football Pools when they met. She had always wanted to be a nurse but had to leave grammar school early when her father died and she was required to replace his income. She had two older brothers, both of whom adored her, but only one saw her grow. Tommy, the eldest, joined the millions who died in the carnage of the First World War. The particular tragedy of Tommy's death, if there really can be grades of tragedy, was that he was killed just a few days before the Armistice was signed, and when he and his mother thought he was safe. The boy soldier, my uncle Tommy, was strolling through a farmyard in France, rifle down, chatting to his friends. In the dark of the barn lay a wounded German soldier, rifle aimed at the door: confused, shivering with cold, and terrified. It was Tommy who had the misfortune to open the door of the barn. He died from a single shot released from the gloom and seconds before his hapless executioner was similarly despatched by his comrades. Two young lives lost: so near to going home, two weeks away from their future. I learned these details from the beautifully handwritten letter crafted for my grandmother by an army chaplain. The news of Tommy's death however did not reach Liverpool until after the Armistice had been signed. Until after my mother's father had swung her in the air yelling 'Thank God' her big brother was coming home. Until after the street party. They never recovered. Grandfather, who had left Blackrock orphanage in Dublin no more than a child to travel unaccompanied to Liverpool, died a few years later. Grandmother died immediately but carried on living.

The chaplain's letter ended with a description of where to find his body, should any member of this poor Irish immigrant family ever find themselves abroad without another war. With a combination of thoughtfulness and efficiency he described Tommy lying under the fifth apple tree on the left as you entered the yard of the farm. I would have loved to think of Tommy sleeping for eternity in the tranquillity of a Belgian farmyard. But no. Pinned to the back of the chaplain's letter, found in the possessions of his younger brother Gerard when he died many years later, was a typed note from the War Office. The scale of the slaughter and the indifference of the authorities were each manifest on that yellowing page. Tommy's name and number had been written into the standard template of a short official letter telling my grandparents that the body of this private soldier, their beloved son, had been moved to a military cemetery in Belgium. The number of his grave was given; it had seven digits. Nothing else. No words of comfort. They'd dug Tommy up and replanted him. If you go to Tommy's grave, please place a stone in remembrance. Read the inscription that my grandparents requested. 'Father forgive them, for they know not what they do.'

When the Second World War broke out my father was called up to the Royal Air Force and trained as a rigger, a member of the ground crew. He told me that he loved the rural locations of the air bases but missed my mother and his new baby, my brother, to the point it made him ill. My mother and brother Brian lived at 2 Forfar Rd while my father was in the RAF. Each night when the air raids came, she packed all her important documents into a small brown suitcase and with Brian in her other arm made her way to the Anderson shelter at the bottom of the garden. One night unknown officials decided the safest way to protect an ammunition train bound for the docks was to shunt it into a residential area, stretching it over the railway bridge a hundred yards or so from where they slept. It took a direct hit from a stray bomb, and the conflagration was such that the house fell onto the Anderson shelter and buried them until they could be dug out later the next day. My mother hugged her baby and waited in the dark to be rescued. Her best friend and her husband had heard of it all on the wireless and assumed they were dead. The city was in chaos, with no means of transport. Nevertheless, she and her husband, home on leave from the army, walked across the city to where the house lay in ruins, expecting confirmation of the terrible news they would have to tell my father. When they got there, they found the fire service had screwed a long pipe through the rubble and into the shelter. Deep inside, mum and Brian held their mouths to the end of it, gulping air and talking to the men who had minutes before thought they were dead. They were the only people in the street to survive; number 2, the first house and farthest from the train. The memory of her friend's voice coming down the tube and the image of his army boots seen through the pipe stayed with my mum forever.

My father was let home on compassionate leave. He told me that when he went to the remains of the house, my mother refused to scrabble for keepsakes or salvage. With the battered brown suitcase in one arm and Brian in the other, she turned to him and said 'We are safe. We still have each other. That's all we need.' And with that she turned and picked her way over the rubble of her newlyweds' home, the glass of the wedding presents crunching under her heels. The experience left its mark. In later years she told me that for a while she thought she was invincible. She would ignore air raid warnings. Rather than move away, she and her mother rented a house on the banks of the Mersey, just over the river in Seaforth. Nobody wanted to live there – it was too near the river and docks – but it was cheap. One night while ignoring yet another air raid warning, she and Brian were caught in the open by the side of the river. Bombs began dropping into the river beside them and for the first time since that terrible night, my mum became scared. She told me much later in life that she said to herself that while she might play Russian roulette with her own life, she had no right to do so with her child's. She managed to run home safely and never took unnecessary risks again.

There were two other legacies of the German air raid on Forfar road. The first was that we couldn't have balloons at parties. The fear of an unexpected bang from a balloon provoked so much anxiety in my mother, and the pain in her face when it burst was so great, that it just wasn't worth it. At the time I was resentful at the lack of balloons at my parties, but if I knew then what I know now I would have felt differently. The second, was the birth of my brother Michael when nine months later my mother found herself going into labour in the middle of yet another air raid. The hospital to which she was admitted took a hit, and with her new baby still wet and wrapped in a blanket, mother and baby were laid on the floor of the hospital laundry van and driven through the blackout to a place of relative safety. If there was a theme to my mother's long and varied life, it was to always count your blessings. Laid next to her was another new mother whose husband had recently perished on HMS Hood. Together in the dark, with the bombs still falling and the van slowly picking its way through the night, they contemplated very different futures.

My father was demobbed from the RAF to work in the Avro Aircraft factory near Oldham. As luck would have it, acquaintances in Liverpool knew of a couple who had a house in Failsworth, not too far from the factory, who would rent it to my mum and dad. Sooner than expected they were reunited and made Failsworth their home till they died. Our landlords were good, kind people who helped rather than exploited their poor tenants. They never increased the rent. Not once over the twenty-five years my parents rented. When 'Uncle Fred' wished to divest himself of the property, he sold it to my parents for the price he had paid all those years ago.

When my eldest sister Stephanie was born, my father was out of the RAF and into work on the markets. He would pick up carpet oddments, sew them together and sell them as carpets in a community that was all make do and mend. As innovative and entrepreneurial as this was, it did not make for luxury. Stephanie's first winter on earth was very nearly her last. She contracted pneumonia and would have died if not for the coalman and the doctor. The former gave free coal 'for the baby's room' for the duration of her illness, and the latter persuaded someone somewhere that she warranted the new wonder drug, 'M&B', that we learned later to call penicillin.

By the time Mary was born, my father had found work as a painter and decorator. He had no training but talked himself into work and learned on the job. He went where the money was to support his growing family, which meant following the dirt and the danger: painting pylons and industrial plants. The wages were meagre, but by working overtime into the evenings and seven days of every week he made sure we got by. Just. We lived in a house so cold in winter, and with the only means of heat a coal fire in one of the downstairs rooms, that my father would resort to lifting the mat from the lino on my bedroom floor and wrapping me in it over the thin bedclothes to help me get to sleep. But equally by now my father no longer had to lift Michael over the gas works' wall to scavenge the coal that had fallen off the delivery trucks.

Then I came along, and after me another baby, Bernadette, to make us a family of six children. It should have been seven. Mum lost baby Dominic in the final weeks of her pregnancy and suffered a loss far deeper and longer lasting than anyone then realised.

How we all lived in that little house is hard to imagine now. When we left, the house appeared to shrink. Where did we all fit? It wasn't just the six kids. When baby Stephanie was so very ill, my father's unmarried sister came to stay to help and never left. Things were helped a little by Brian, like my father before him, going away to be a priest (and, like my father, later rejecting it). However, we did later take in an unofficial foster child, so things got back to usual. Space was also created by Auntie Mary my father's sister living with us, taking Bernadette and I to Liverpool each weekend to stay with my father's other surviving sister, Auntie Frances. Nevertheless, it took some juggling and some imagination on my mother's part to keep the peace, and the social workers at bay. We all shared rooms, obviously, but the pattern of occupation was constantly changing as one after another we each passed through puberty. An innocent passing remark about a sibling's changing anatomy was all that was required to trigger a reshuffle.

Spending weekends with Auntie Frances was no hardship. It was magical, for Bernadette and I had time alone with Auntie Mary who we both loved to distraction. Free from being torn between loyalty to our proper mum and the deep bond we had forged with the woman who basically brought us up, we could indulge ourselves and bask in the warmth of her undivided attention. Auntie Mary loved these times too, alone with two small children she treated as her own, until Friday evening turned into Sunday night, and we caught the bus back home to Failsworth.

Auntie Frances had been a missionary nun in Borneo when the Second World War broke out and she was captured by the Japanese. She was starved and beaten, and whatever else they did to her, it made her turn her back on religious service when she was liberated from Kuching POW Camp by the Australians. I found out later that she features in the book of the wartime experiences of Agnes Newton Keith, a fellow prisoner of war. In that book, *Three Came Home*, she refers to a Sister Stephanie, the religious name of my Auntie Frances, and the name given to my sister when my parents found out that Auntie Frances had survived. In that book the author describes that, however hard the inmates suffered, particularly with their lack of food, the nuns suffered more and gave much of what little rations they had to the children. When she was brought back to Manchester in a hospital train, my brother Brian says he ran screaming from the carriage, shouting that there was a skeleton in the bed. When she recovered, she left the order, trained as a midwife in what is now the North Manchester General Hospital, married, and became a district midwife in a very poor part of

Liverpool, very much as portrayed in the BBC television series Call the Midwife. We didn't have a telephone at home until my mid-teens but Auntie Frances had two, one of which was by her bed. In the dark quiet of the night I would hear the phone ring and picture Auntie Frances slipping from her bed and into the dark cold streets of Liverpool. In the morning, seemingly entirely unaffected by her lack of sleep, she would excitedly tell me all about the latest addition to the post-war baby boom. After breakfast, she would put on her blue gabardine and nurse's hat, and together we would set off to review her night's work. Walking proudly by her side and carrying her medical bag, I beamed as men tipped their caps, women said 'Morning Sister Gannon', and demonstrated to me how, like me, they loved my aunt and the wonderful work that she did. On arriving at the house, I was always struck by the smell of new baby and the cosiness and peace that descended on a house after birth. In a very different age, as my midwife aunt went upon her rounds, no one seemed to bother about the little boy who accompanied her; welcoming me into the house, showing me the new baby, and feeding me biscuits in the kitchen while she examined the mother in private , behind a blanket hung over a line.

Life had a rhythm and security that still glows in my memory. It couldn't last, and it didn't. Auntie Mary died; three of us children got TB; and my father fell off a roof at work and was badly injured. Things would never be the same again.

She'd been ill for a while but didn't see the doctor. She was always regarded as old, and I suppose just allowed to slip away, but I was shocked years later when the inscription on the gravestone truly registered. She was only in her sixties. Younger than I am today. She was left to die in her bed, without any discussion of hospital or specialists, and without any treatment to speak of. Actually, she didn't die in her bed. She died in Stephanie's bed. Auntie Mary never had a bed. She slept downstairs on a bed settee when everyone else had gone upstairs. She rose while the house still slept and lit the fire. On freezing winter mornings, I only had to run downstairs to her still warm bedclothes and snuggle under while she dressed me under the covers with clothes she'd already warmed by the fire. I knew something serious was happening therefore when I came home from school and she was in my sister's bed. Her GP wasn't ours. For some reason she had another one and looking back, being as generous as I can be, perhaps not a very good one. She couldn't breathe, and when my mother asked him what could be done, he wrote out a prescription. He left the slip of paper on the dressing table and left. My mother was simply too respectful of authority, and doctors especially, to ask any further questions.

I was a somewhat precocious child and mum relied on me for a lot of practical things as my father was always out at work. So, it was not unusual that my mother would ask me to take a prescription the half mile to the local chemist. When I got to the chemists, the pharmacist looked down at me, not only from his height behind the counter, but I sensed also with the contempt he held for me and my ilk: a family that that would send a boy of barely ten for a prescription, let alone for one like this. 'You'll never manage,' he said. 'Of course I will,' I said, with the stubbornness in the face of authority that would dog me for the rest of my life. 'So be it' he said, and slowly rolled out an enormous metal cylinder from behind the counter. It towered above my head.

The prescription was for oxygen. The look on his face was triumphant. I went to the gas cylinder and tried to move it. It was surprisingly cold, and the heaviest thing I'd ever tried to lift. People in the shop sniggered and the pharmacist talked to them over my head in a 'well what do you expect' kind of way. It still wouldn't budge, and nearly fell on top of me. I could feel the pressure it exerted on the wooden floor. I ran out of the shop, my face burning red with anger. I didn't cry. I was blazing and humiliated. I didn't want my mother to worry though. She wouldn't know what to do with the oxygen cylinder, any more than I did, and I wasn't going to let him treat her like he'd treated me. As I ran home, I hatched a plan. Behind the shed were the remains of Bernadette's old pram. We children had been saving it to use the wheels to build a wooden go-cart, or bogey as we called them. Without mum noticing, I slipped by the side of the house, got hold of the battered pram, and ran back to the chemist's shop. I couldn't get the pram up the steps and through the door but opened the door enough for the pharmacist to see my proposed solution. He looked. I stood. For a few minutes I thought he'd turn away, but he didn't. He slowly rolled the heavy cylinder to the door and tipped it sideways over the steps and onto the pram. The springs buckled and collapsed so far down that I thought the pram must surely disintegrate. But it held, and without comment or looking back, he simply closed the door. I tried to push the pram, but it wouldn't move. I was not going to give up now, and I was not going to let the pharmacist be witness to my defeat and further humiliation. And more than that, I had to do it for Auntie Mary. I leant against the handles of the pram until I was almost horizontal and pushed and pushed until, slowly but surely, the pram began to move. Now my problems really started. The weight of the cylinder caused the pram to rock and roll like a thing demented and its momentum meant I couldn't really stop it without crashing. It almost bounced off several times, and if it had, I knew all would have been lost. Without help I could never have got it back on. Some grownups looked at me with apparent concern. Some shook their heads in contempt, others simply laughed, but nobody offered to help. But I got it home.

My mother, somewhat taken aback, asked the man next door to help us carry it upstairs and we were eventually able to stand it next to Auntie Mary's bed. But what now? The pharmacist had dropped a bag into the pram as he closed the door. I recognised an oxygen cylinder from watching hospital dramas on the television and I knew to place the mask I found inside the bag over Auntie Mary's mouth. She was sweating and her damp head lolled backwards and forwards in my arms as I secured it by pulling the elastic around the back of her head. She could hardly speak but smiled so gratefully and whispered huskily 'thank you, son.' She always called me her son. I twiddled with the knob, but nothing happened. Auntie Mary's life depended on me and I'd failed. Surely it must be working. Mum and I convinced ourselves that we could hear a hissing of gas and Auntie Mary said it made her feel better. But we knew deep down it didn't. When my brother Michael came home, he told me to go back to the chemist and get the valve opener. I felt so bad. Such an ignorant failure. I ran all the way back to the chemists and burst through the door. The pharmacist didn't look surprised; he was expecting me. He held up the valve opener and simply said, 'You'll be wanting this I expect.' I wish I had said then all that I would say now. But I had to get it back to Auntie Mary as quickly as my aching little legs would let me. I took it in silence and ran back all the way home, where Michael opened the valve and we listened with joy to the now unmistakable hissing of the gas.

Auntie Mary died a few days later. I never went into that shop again. My rage was replaced by grief, and as I grew and learned more of the world, I recognised the shallowness and insecurities behind his feelings of superiority. I also vowed to try my best to never treat anyone like that, and to never be the one to pass by the little boy struggling with a huge oxygen cylinder bouncing on and off a battered old pram, without stopping to offer help.

Losing my Auntie Mary was like losing my mother. The fact that I still had a mother confused and distressed me, and the depth of my grief was never acknowledged. I played with a football alone in the street after her funeral, hating myself for living on when I could never have conceived of life without her. But here was life without her, and I'd let her down. Things would never be the same. It seems to me now that Auntie Mary died of TB. Nursing her so closely was my undoing. Not too long after she died, when Auntie Frances was visiting she told my mum that the pains in my chest were serious, and she should get the doctor. My GP was in a different class altogether from Auntie Mary's GP. The sort of doctor I have tried to be during my career. When as a new consultant after I gave a guest lecture at the local hospital near to where I was brought up, the room was opened up to questions. Overcome with almost parental pride and excitement, Dr Cresswell stood up immediately, and to my embarrassment told the audience that he'd delivered me. He didn't tell them that without him I wouldn't be there. That he'd saved my life when, over twenty years before, he had examined me on Auntie Mary's bed settee, tapped my chest, and used the phone at the corner shop to call the ambulance. No blue lights then, just a tinny bell ringing through the streets and my poor mother looking at me with such worry that I thought my heart would break. At the hospital they drained fluid from my chest, did a lumbar puncture, and placed a tube in my stomach. TB was diagnosed and I got worse and became very ill indeed. Another lumbar puncture followed, and I expect they thought I may have had TB meningitis.

I was put into an isolation cubicle where I was to learn that the boy in the cubicle next to me died. The parish priest came to see me, and I believe I had the last rites. Public health officials discovered that my brother Michael, then my sister Mary, had now also contracted TB. They were each sent to a sanatorium for over a year. I learned later of the humiliation felt by my mother when the authorities one by one inspected her home, knowing full well the association of TB with our poverty and overcrowding.

One by one we all returned home. Michael married and Mary tried to pick up the schooling she'd lost. It seemed like a lifetime before I finally re-joined my classmates for that all-important eleven-plus year. On my first day back, on entering the playground, I found myself surrounded by all my classmates. Rather than the applause for surviving I momentarily fantasised I was about to receive, a girl, nominated by them for the task, stepped forwards, and without warning, slapped me across my face. Hard. She announced to the crowd, in the manner of a public prosecutor, that I was dirty, and that because of me, they'd all had to have injections. My mother had never mentioned the word TB to me, only pleurisy. I remember now how I neither flinched nor cried. I stood firm and silent. The crowd too fell silent, and not now knowing what else to do, drifted away. I went into class and never looked back.

As a family, though, we were still not quite done with social workers. One afternoon, not long after my return to school, I came home to find mum in tears in the kitchen. 'Go upstairs and talk to your father. He's had an accident.' My dad was stood up in the bathroom, shaving. The whole of one leg was in plaster. He looked so vulnerable. He'd been painting a roof, fell off and badly fractured his lower leg and ankle. He was off work a long time and could never again earn the 'danger money' for working at heights. Without my dad's weekly wage, we were in serious trouble. We owned nothing outright; everything we had was on hire purchase and much of it owed to a tallyman who came every week for his money. My mum swallowed her pride and asked the woman in the shop two streets away for a job behind the counter. This kept us going, and the social workers at bay. I of course never knew about the social workers at the time. It was my brother Michael who told me many years later just how close we came to being taken into care. But eventually my father recovered enough to find a job as a maintenance painter in a factory.

From the age of fourteen I worked on a market stall selling fruit and veg. Every Saturday in term time and every holiday in between. I never received pocket money and in the world my parents came from, I was a man at fourteen, and should at least in part be supporting myself. On market days I left the house before six in the morning and got home after seven at night. I met the stallholder at the wholesale market in Manchester where I helped him load the wagon. We drove to the market and assembled the stall. We then unloaded the wagon and filled the stall we'd built, and I spent the rest of the day hauling sacks of potatoes and boxes of fruit and veg from the lorry park to the market to keep it filled. Backwards and forwards; in any weather. And at the end of the day we did it all in reverse. It was miserable most of the time, but it earned me money and gave me independence. It broadened my outlook with the range of people I met and worked with, many of whom were not long out of prison – the markets being the only place they could get work without questions being asked. And it probably encouraged the relentless work ethic and physical resilience required later in my career.

Preface

From Grammar School, I made it into Manchester Medical School. When I started, they handed us each a questionnaire to find out, amongst other things, what social background we came from. Social ranking for a long time was from I to V, based on your father's or your own occupation. Doctors were social class I; I was social class V. When the results were fed back to us, we were informed that the distribution of social classes in my academic year, in the autumn of 1970, differed little, if at all, from that sixty years previously, just before the First World War.

I'd relished the thought of university, the intellectual challenge. However, the anatomy dissection rooms disgusted me. The smell of formalin and the running fat of the corpses in the heat of summer made me physically sick. At the end of my first year I resolved to leave medical school and become an artist. What sort of artist was never quite clear to me, but the life of a writer or musician seemed equally attractive. At the end of term, I slipped into the house and suggested to my Dad that I take him for a pint. In the pub I opened up to him about my ambition to be an artist – a writer or maybe a musician. 'Good for you,' he said. 'Many famous artists and writers were doctors. Look at A. J. Cronin. Look at Somerset Maugham.' 'Mind you,' he added, almost distractedly, 'they did qualify first. But no matter.' I began to breathe easier. With each artist, poet, and writer with any medical connection that he brought to the table over the course of the evening, he gently added the rider that they'd at least first qualified. He said he thought it was the most sophisticated thing in the world to qualify as a doctor and then turn away, never practise, and dedicate yourself to your art. So we hatched a plan, a secret plan, to be known only to us two. I would from now on be an artist, a musician, but it was to be a secret. I'd beat them at their own game. I'd qualify then run away. What a plan. What a man. We hugged and made our way home. As we opened the door, he said 'please don't tell your mother, son.'

It was there as a medical student I was to diagnose my father's terminal illness and break the news to my family of what was to come. He just about hung on to see me graduate but died shortly afterwards. Immediately after the ceremony, my now terminally ill father took me to one side. Looking at me in my cap and gown he reminded me of that day when we talked about me being an artist, and how I'd wanted to leave the University. I had to confess to him that it had now somewhat faded a little from my memory. 'I remember it well,' he said. 'I've held my breath for five years. I knew if a said anything even slightly wrong you might actually go ahead with it, give up the best chance you would ever have to break out.' He was so thin and weak by then, but he smiled, and I blushed. I loved my dad.

By the time I graduated I was far more at ease with my self-image. Not that newly qualified doctors automatically take on the mantle (or stethoscope) with ease, but I was no more or less comfortable with my new role and status in life than the next. Social class V to social class I in a day. An Apollo rocket couldn't have moved faster. I'd left home once I went to university, and didn't go back to Failsworth, other than to visit. Not until we children all moved back home to look after our mum in her own final days.

I was a consultant in emergency medicine when I rang my mother to tell her that I was going into hospital for an endoscopy and not to worry. Before I could, she revealed she had been meaning to ring me to ask my advice about the difficulty in swallowing she was experiencing. As she unfolded to me about her symptoms, I knew sadly what it was likely to be. As it turned out, my worst fears were confirmed, and in a bizarre twist of fate my endoscopy showed I too had the early signs of what she was about to die from, although I managed to keep my surgery and diagnosis from her and my family until after her death. I was at the start of a series of surgical operations and an additional unfolding chronic illness, but it was imperative now that everyone's attention was on her, and our desire to honour her final wishes of dying at home, in her own bed, and surrounded by her family. The little house that seemed to have shrunk so tiny in our absence, now grew back to accommodate us all as we returned to be with her in her final days. All our newly acquired identities slipped quietly into the background as we spent the weeks of her final summer gently laughing with our mum, as day by day she weakened, then died.

For all the relative hardships of my early life, I was blessed with knowing love, and seeing people around me trying their best to be, and to do, good. Although I was brought up in a religious family, I do not have religion now; abandoned long ago, and as soon as I left home. But all that I have admired in those around me – their goodness, their kindness, the giving of themselves – can, and for me should, be done regardless, simply for its own sake. Suffering must be relieved wherever it may be found.

1.

Lockdown

Kosovo / Manchester / Sarajevo / Sierra Leone

I would conclude my career as a practising doctor in the city where it all started – Manchester – some fifty years after starting medical school. In December 2019, an outbreak of a new corona virus was reported in the city of Wuhan, in South Eastern China. In a densely populated city of over 10 million people, the disease spread rapidly. With 1500 flights a year between the UK with China, it didn't take long for it to spread here, and on 31 January 2020 the first two cases of what was now called Covid-19 were confirmed on these shores. Less than two months later, as the number of cases rapidly increased, the Prime Minister announced to the nation that we should 'Stay at home. Protect the NHS. Save lives.' We were now in lockdown. Such was the concern that the National Health Service (NHS) might be rapidly overwhelmed, a number of emergency 'field hospitals', to be known as the Nightingale Hospitals, were to be rapidly assembled across the country. Having recently retired from the University, doing only intermittent consultant and advisory work, I was looking forward to a quieter life. It wasn't to be. Having begun my career in emergency and disaster medicine here in Manchester, I was moved to be asked to bring home the experience of a lifetime to the aid of a city, my city, embroiled in the greatest public health emergency of the last 100 years and an unfolding national disaster. I suddenly found myself the Medical Director of the NHS Nightingale Hospital in the North West of England. We pulled a team together, built and staffed a 650-bed hospital from scratch, and opened it to patients in just two weeks. This, though, was not the first Field Hospital that I'd built.

I have spent a lifetime responding to disasters, whether caused by 'natural' events such as earthquakes, or the wholly unnatural and inhuman disaster that is war. The thread that binds them and pulled me towards them is the overwhelming of healthcare facilities, and a failure to cope. In sudden onset disasters, it is too often the result of a failure to prepare that heralds the failure to cope. There are natural phenomena of course, like earthquakes for example, but the disaster that follows them is not of itself necessarily 'natural'; something that is always inevitable. The buildings that fell on top of people did not always have to fall; they could, or should, have been made strong enough to stay up. The first earthquake I ever responded to was in Armenia in 1988. Over 25,000 people perished as buildings crumbled and walls fell, crushing to death those inside and on the streets below. Only a year later, an even stronger earthquake struck Palo Alto in California. Only sixty-three citizens of the richest state in the richest country in the world perished, saved not by nature but by wealth and the architecture it can buy. There is too often a failure to build to the required standard, sometimes from neglect, but usually for lack of money. People, countries, simply cannot afford to build their dwellings far enough away from the hazards they know they will face, or strong enough to withstand them.

*

The site chosen for the hospital was the Manchester Central Conference Centre. I knew it in its original glory as the Manchester Central Railway Station. A magnificent piece of Victorian railway architecture, where a huge arc of iron and glass curved over both passengers and platforms beneath. As a small child I had taken my first railway journey from there. The 'boat train' left Manchester Central for Holyhead, where it lined up on the quayside beside gangways taking passengers in a couple of steps onto the ferry to Ireland. And it was a steam train. The smoke from its firebox spread all around the station's huge confines – at first up into the air, and then down and all around. Some sixty years later I would look again at this continuous open space, with its high vaulted ceiling and know, that just as the smoke could not be contained or stay in one area, neither could an airborne virus.

*

An outbreak of disease is usually a natural phenomenon, and a pandemic of a new virus could challenge most countries' ability to cope. But not all, and not all to the same extent or for as long. At the time of writing, the United Kingdom is towards the bottom of the international response league and at the top of deaths per million population. This public health, social and economic disaster cannot be dismissed or excused as a 'natural disaster.' The UK's ability to cope was fatally undermined by a failure to prepare. Add to this the systematic degradation of the NHS and public health capacity over the preceding years, and a failure to mount a timely and comprehensive response, and it is easy to see why we have fared particularly badly. In the Global Health Security Index of 195 nations assessing how well a state's health care system would 'treat the sick and protect health workers', the UK fell from second to being one of the most vulnerable countries in the world. It's not as though we hadn't been warned. As recently as 2016, the UK ran a pandemic simulation exercise, codenamed 'Cygnus', which showed clearly that the UK had a critical shortage of ventilators and personal protective equipment (PPE). But nothing was done. Even when the pandemic was upon us, when WHO urged all nations to institute a policy of 'Test, Trace and Isolate', again not enough was done. England's Deputy Chief Medical Officer went so far as to argue that it wasn't needed, that we were somehow exceptional: 'The clue with WHO is in its title – it's a *World* Health Organisation,' she explained during a Downing Street press briefing. 'And it is addressing all countries across the world, with entirely different health infrastructures.'[1] True, but our infrastructure had by then been fatally degraded.

Planning is everything. And in every field hospital, but particularly in this one, infection prevention and control, IPC, would be front and centre to planning and practice. No surprise then that our first appointment was a Director of Infection Prevention and Control. For set-up we recruited a specialist in IPC from Manchester-based UK-Med, the charity I established over thirty years ago and an organisation experienced in infection control in outbreaks of disease, including the ebola virus in West Africa.

UK-Med itself grew out of my work in emergency medicine, first in the UK, then internationally.

On moving to a new post as Consultant in Manchester in 1987, I was asked to address a specific problem. A child had recently been impaled on railings that had penetrated the back of his head, and in spite of his proximity to several hospitals, there was no-one with the right skills free to leave the hospital immediately and remove him from his gibbet. There followed a painful and distressing delay, played out in the glare of local media, until someone of sufficient experience could attend. The child lived, and as far as I know made a good recovery. The affair prompted the Chair of the Health Authority to phone me immediately after my appointment, and even before I took up my post, describing the problem and telling me to find a solution. They would support me in every way, give me everything I needed – except, of course, money. The answer, to my mind, lay in recruiting a team of senior, experienced nurses and doctors to volunteer in their off-duty time, and be available, 24 hours a day, in support of the emergency services. Given the lack of financial support, their contribution would have to be voluntary. So, we raised the money ourselves; enough to both equip and maintain the team, the new South Manchester Accident Rescue Team, SMART. We were also given the money by well-wishers to buy an ambulance, state of the art communications equipment, and fire and chemical proof clothing for each team member. And so, the concept behind much of my future work was born: (1) Recruit highly skilled volunteers; (2) Raise money to train and equip them to work in a difficult environment; (3) Place them on a register that guarantees a team is available to deploy, wherever and whenever, it is required. When not on call for the team, they were in their day job, usually in the NHS, treating patients and maintaining and honing their skills. It worked in Manchester, and as we expanded and established a national UK-Med team, it has continued to work nationally, and then internationally, now allowing expert medical support to be deployed from the UK to humanitarian emergencies around the world.[2]

The shared emotional uplift from coming together in a common cause is powerful and binds we humans together. I have never had difficulty in recruiting volunteers to my teams, whether it involves leaving your bed in the cold and dark of a winter's night to help the victims of road traffic collisions in Manchester, or stepping up to volunteer to travel into danger overseas to help the victims of wars, earthquakes and disease. And so it was with the Nightingale, As the Covid-19 pandemic wreaked its havoc, people stepped up, came out of retirement, changed jobs, moved cities, all to help those most in need.

The rapid hospital build was the combined effort of many groups, organisations, and individuals. But the kick start, the key element that got us off the ground and running, was the experience of those who had done it before. Five years earlier, UK-Med had recruited, trained, and deployed medical staff, largely from the NHS, into an ebola treatment centre in Kerrytown in Sierra Leone, built in a few short weeks by the British Army. That expertise carried over in the institutional memories of both organisations, and in the abilities of those who had worked there.

*

In lockdown everyone was required to stay in their home to limit the spread of the virus. I have been in lockdown before; not to avoid an epidemic of disease, but an epidemic of violence. Venturing out of one's house in the siege of Sarajevo was to balance the risk of being shot by a sniper against how important it was for you to leave the relative safety of your home. Staying in was no guarantee of safety either, as mortar and tank shells fell indiscriminately, but the chances of death when staying inside were less. The analogy with Covid-19 is a little stretched, but not altogether farfetched – we were still balancing the risks of going out against staying indoors, most noticeably at the start, even if the odds were stacked a little differently. We were all rightly frightened and there was a real choice to be made between how much you really wanted something and the risks you were prepared to take to get it. The Covid lockdowns have been measured in months, rather than the years it took for the siege of Sarajevo to end. Nevertheless, every day I am reminded of the constant tension that persisting threat and uncertainty can bring. Of the desire to break out.

I think of the day in Sarajevo when a middle-aged woman could take the lockdown no longer, and left the relative safety of her enclosed darkened inner room to stand in the morning light, breathe the air of an open window, and fill a kettle for a much-wanted pot of coffee. A Serbian tank commander in the nearby hills saw her through his binoculars – kettle in hand, tap water running – and without hesitation, care, or mercy, fired his shell directly at her. I met her in the operating theatre: arms and legs blown off, sucking air through a gaping hole in her chest, slowly gasping her final breaths.

*

I'd built a pop-up hospital before, with the help of the British Army and this time in Kosovo, shortly after NATO intervened in the conflict there between the ethnic Albanians and the ethnic Serbs. I had been asked by the British Government to assist in the immediate post-conflict recovery, and specifically, in the restoration of the major teaching hospital in the capital of Kosovo, Pristina. Before leaving Kosovo, the Serbs had completely trashed the hospital – smashing every sink, removing every light bulb, destroying everything they couldn't carry. They left the bodies in the mortuary, though, having first turned off the power to the refrigerators. In the sweltering heat of a Kosovan summer, corpses had partially liquefied. They'd also left the doors open, and packs of feral dogs were now dragging body parts from the mortuary and across the hospital grounds. Not all were parts: one dog was standing over a baby. In one of the most heroic and selfless acts of human kindness I've been proud to witness, the British Army gathered all the remains together, and placed them into body bags. The mortuary was cleansed of its human detritus by young men and women, working in appalling conditions; quietly, methodically, restoring a semblance of dignity to the dead of a foreign war.

Against this backdrop of chaos and violence, with pockets of gunfire still bursting out around the hospital site, we set out to establish an essential emergency healthcare service to Pristina, and by extension to Kosovo. We couldn't do everything at once, so where to begin? We certainly had to treat injuries from gunshot wounds, landmines, and cluster bombs, let alone the casualties from lawless driving in a lawless country. We would need to ensure women were delivered safely of their babies and caesarean sections made available to them if required. And people would still be falling ill. We'd identified the least damaged building, which we planned to convert into an Emergency Centre. By a stroke of extreme good luck, an old friend and colleague (now Surgeon General) Tim Hodgetts was posted to Kosovo at that time, and as I pondered how we might set about our task, he sought me out and calmly revealed that he had upon his person a set of plans for such an eventuality. So British Army, Crown Agents[3] and Kosovar engineers gutted, refurbished and equipped the building. There we built an operating theatre and an emergency room where the acutely ill and injured could be received and resuscitated. We also built an intensive care unit where the sickest could be cared for, and a pharmacy to safely receive, store and dispense essential drugs. And all in a matter of weeks.

The department was opened by the then Secretary of State for International Development, Clare Short. A large red sign, written in English, identified it as the Emergency Centre. Why English? The Serbs had told me that it must be in Serbian: Kosovo was part of Serbia. If it was in Albanian, they would blow up the centre. The Albanians had told me that if it was in Serbian, they too would blow it up. So English it was. When I revisited some years later, both the sign and the building had remained intact.

The same can-do attitude fired up all the volunteers at the Nightingale hospital we built. Much of what has been removed from the NHS was replaced. Professionals were allowed an independence hitherto eroded or lost altogether, management was accessible and light touch, and hierarchies were flattened. Staff and patients reported being valued and well cared for and the altruism that lies at the heart of the NHS was allowed to flourish. The NHS Nightingale Northwest was an enormously rewarding place to work. When people step up as volunteers, they are clearly already motivated, and leadership is no burden. When they step up and into the unknown, into potential danger, there is a common bond and mutual support that is truly uplifting.

*

But as in any deployment anywhere in the world, there are always internal and external forces that criticise, undermine or seek to thwart what you are doing. As my work at the Nightingale unfolded, I realised this would be no different. Covid-19 in the UK, or certainly in England, played out against a backdrop of a near catastrophic failure of the British government, first to heed the warnings about a pandemic that was inevitable and foretold, and then respond to it appropriately and in a timely fashion. An unjustified exceptionalism, coupled with a slavish commitment to outsourcing hitherto government-run public services to private companies with little or no previous relevant experience, meant that when we came to venture out from our lockdown bunkers into the gunsights of the virus, it was without the covering fire of a comprehensive test, trace and isolate programme.

In my international work I have at times found one arm of the British government pushing me forwards, while another arm was pulling me back. So it was at the Nightingale. One part of the NHS was happy for us to expand, while another was putting on the brakes. And to this heady mix was added the new quasi-religious adherence to the 'business model' of healthcare delivery. A misnomer if ever there was one, as we are not selling anything – it's already been bought by the taxpayer – but has led everything to be outsourced, as far as it can be. The NHS has been privatised in plain sight. It's now McNHS, with the blue logo of the NHS in place of the golden arches – appearing to unify what is essentially a group of individual businesses. So when the Nightingales were launched, irrespective of the expertise on hand and the gravity of the emergency in which we found ourselves, the dogma was that everything should be outsourced and was up for grabs. That dictated that a private consultancy firm should be inserted into the matrix, just as they were in the disastrous test, trace and isolate debacle. A parallel structure, and one with limited, if any, medical expertise. I can see the value to the consultancy of this arrangement, not only in financial terms (some of their senior staff were prepared to charge the NHS £3,000 per day plus VAT), but also in the opportunity to glean intelligence and data from working close to clinicians. But its value to the NHS and to the patient, is much less clear.

*

After 100 days or more of the first lockdown, we were allowed to venture out from our bunkers, if only for a while. People had taken seriously the government advice to stay away from hospitals, as much out of fear as duty, while the NHS gave itself over almost entirely to the virus. And as happened in Sierra Leone during the Ebola outbreak, when a response blinkered to everything besides the one issue allowed the number of women dying in childbirth to rise catastrophically, so possibly here also, too much other suffering went unseen, unheard and unnoticed..

Building a field hospital in the UK, and particularly within the NHS, was always going to be high risk. The rapid build of a clinical facility in a building designed for something else entirely would make it difficult to maintain normal infection prevention and control procedures, made even more challenging by its very purpose being to care for those with an already highly infectious virus, about which we still knew relatively little. Added to this was the need to garner an additional workforce without draining the local NHS and to ensure that such a disparate group of volunteers could be trained and supervised to provide the care needed and to the right standard. I knew too that, irrespective of the 'Field Hospital' soubriquet, in practice the public and political tolerance for any shortcomings would be low. But we managed, and we managed well. A herculean effort by a team brought together almost overnight ensured that patients received good and safe care; that wards and everywhere in the building were always cleaned rigorously; that access to areas of infection was controlled; and staff were trained in the use of personal protective equipment (PPE) and provided with it at all times.

So why did we all take the personal and professional risks of stepping forward into the unknown? Well, there was a clear national emergency and just how much the NHS would be threatened by its consequences remained unclear when we were asked. In my view, building a national insurance policy of additional beds was entirely reasonable. That they should all have been intensive care beds was logical given what was known at the time, and the experience of other countries. What was not anticipated was the almost complete repurposing of the NHS to combat one disease. Bed capacity was increased. Extra staffing for these beds was facilitated by the redeployment of staff from those areas now idle. Almost all other work ground down to a halt. The third factor in the conundrum of how the NHS coped against the odds was the response of the public. Until the Prime Minister's adviser Dominic Cummings, broke his own rules and made a now infamous trip to Durham, there was remarkable adherence to the lockdown. Patients stayed away from activities that would normally book their ticket to hospital, such as drunkenness and road traffic collisions, and a widespread and well founded fear of contracting the infection in hospitals, led people with other medical conditions to stay away. By the end of the two weeks it took to build the hospital, we knew that the 650 beds we had equipped would not be needed at that point in time, but we did not know enough to be certain that it wouldn't be needed at all. So, we opened.

Our first patient arrived on the day we opened and we continued to receive patients over the three months that we were first open. There was a persistent dilemma for those wishing to refer patients. If there was an overwhelming pandemic, and the NHS was on its knees, then sending someone to a field hospital, often some distance away, was justified: there was simply no alternative. But with bed capacity holding up, it was difficult for many clinicians to be sure it was always in their patent's best interests to move them into a temporary facility. We knew that the level of care we could offer, with our high staff patient ratio and specialist rehabilitation teams, no longer really qualified us as a field hospital, and for many patients a move to the Nightingale might very well be in their best interests – but it was not our call to make. As the NHS gradually reopened the Nightingale Hospital was moved into standby, ready to reactivate, fully equipped, with all its policies in place, providing the insurance policy as was first intended. And reopen it did a few months later, but in a different guise. This time as a community led facility to facilitate an earlier discharge of non-Covid elderly patients. It was led by general practitioners and allied healthcare professionals, though I continued to act in an advisory capacity until the end of March 2021 when it closed completely.

*

The Nightingales have been criticised for being a mere gesture; a political folly. They have been caught up in the general disappointment and anger at the perceived incompetence of the UK Government's response to the Covid-19 crisis. But the policy was a good one, and I have been glad to play my part. In responding meaningfully to any large-scale emergency (and often in my experience, to any emergency) there must be an initial 'no regrets' policy. Former United States Secretary of State General Colin Powell's operated on a 40/70 principle for decision-making in an emergency. To make a reasonable decision in a rapidly unfolding emergency, you will need at least 40 per cent of the information you would like, but if you wait for 70 per cent or more of the information, it will usually be too late. Events have run on and many of the choices you thought you had are now redundant. And so it was with the Nightingales. Had we waited for all the information we would have liked, then thousands of patients might already have died for want of a hospital bed. It was a risk worth taking.

I've faced similar dilemmas when sending teams to sudden onset disasters overseas. We deploy with a 'no regrets' policy. If we are asked to help and the assessments indicate that we can do some good, then we will go. If, as the catastrophe unfolds, the need for outside help subsides, then we can always go home. As long as we were asked to help, the deployment is justified. There is much good faith to gain from responding to requests and much to lose by refusing.

The response to the Covid pandemic here in the UK has reflected much of the good and the bad I've seen in responding to large scale emergencies over many years. Particularly, the dismissal of some interventions as mere gestures and the rapid upsurge in public support for others. The altruism of those, who despite the risks, uncertainties, and even danger, step forwards, and the venality of those politicians who fail to protect them. Most important is the ever-present conflict between doing the most for the most people and your best for the individual, when demands on resources are so great they may reach saturation point – for example ventilators. But as with some other countries I've operated in, the rationing of resources and intensive care beds in the United Kingdom, is not new, and has not been confined to national emergencies. In one hospital I worked at, the policy was not to take patients over 65 onto the intensive or coronary care units if they had been resuscitated from cardiac arrest elsewhere in the hospital. There was no written rule to this effect and certainly no scientific basis for such action: it was an autonomous decision made by a group of consultants to ration beds to those they considered more deserving. I challenged this, of course. First by confrontation, which was only partially successful, and then by garnering objective evidence. I reviewed the records of almost 750 patients who had suffered a cardiac arrest on the general wards of the hospital. I was able to show that whilst 90% per cent of those aged less than 65 years were transferred to a specialist unit after they had been resuscitated, only half of those older than 65 years were transferred. However, regardless of age, review of the records showed that transfer to a specialist care facility had a significant and positive influence on outcome for everyone. Patients were clearly being unfairly, and indeed unethically, denied life-saving care on an arbitrary basis, and once exposed, it stopped.

Fairness comes in many guises. If we were asked about prioritising patient care in the Covid pandemic from behind what the philosopher John Rawls' refers to as the 'veil of ignorance', blinded to the diagnosis, could we distinguish between the immediate risks to health from the disease itself, and other life-threatening conditions? Could we assess the wider risks to general population health from damage to the economy? In combatting Covid we were inevitably drawn to the threat immediately before us, as we are in any humanitarian crisis. But as soon as possible we must widen our field of vision and distribute resources – and justly. There must always come a point when we can't do everything for everyone, or do it all at the same time, and so must then look to do the most for the most, and prioritise some over others. This is the principle behind triage, and in medicine comes largely from the work of Napoleon's surgeon, Baron Dominique-Jean Larrey, over 200 years ago. In addition to his 'flying ambulances' for the rapid transport of casualties to what were to become the modern-day field hospitals, he most famously looked to sort his patients according to the severity of their injury and the urgency with which they required treatment, and not according to their rank that had hitherto been the norm.

But what do we do when everyone is severely ill or injured, and everybody's care is urgent? To maintain the highest standard of care across a population we may have to engage another tier of triage and alter the level of care to each individual, in so doing seeking to provide the greatest benefit to the greatest number.

The Nightingales were to be reborn at the beginning of 2022 in response to an even more infectious variant of the virus, called Omicron, now as annexes within or immediately alongside existing hospitals. Once again concerns were raised about their appropriateness, but there was potentially a very significant threat. This time too there was the additional issue of an exhausted and chronically diminished workforce. If these new 'mini-Nightingales' were to function, they could only serve as holding bays for patients already on the road to recovery but not yet fit for discharge. They would be given basic care by minimally trained staff, overseen by a small team of fully trained healthcare officials managing a much larger cohort of patients than would usually be the case: a shift towards mass casualty triage that mercifully was not ultimately required.

The pandemic is still not over, as much as our politicians might wish it away. A country once so well prepared has suffered one of the highest death rates in the developed world and whenever it ends, another will follow. So if the promised inquiry into the lessons of Covid delivers anything less than the unvarnished truth, there will inevitably only be more of the same to come in future.

2.

Choices

Manchester / Iran–Iraq Border / Iran

Practising medicine is often about making choices, some of which are hard. I was already making difficult choices before I volunteered to work in disaster stricken and war-ravaged countries around the world, and there were harder ones to come when I did. They remain with me, have affected me deeply and shaped my thinking.

The General Medical Council says that doctors must make the care of their patients their first concern. A superficially simple instruction, but loaded with uncertainty. How do we define care? I might care about my patient, but do I have to do anything? Yes and no. Yes, caring in medicine implies not just feeling, but doing. 'I feel your pain' helps no one. 'I'll relieve your pain' does. But also, no: caring can sometimes mean not doing, standing back, withholding and even withdrawing care. Sometimes 'I'll relieve your pain' might need to be fortified by 'I'll not prolong your pain' and for some even, 'I'll end your pain.' And that is only for the patient before me. What if the patient is not my patient? If the patient in the next bed, or next hospital, is another doctor's patient and needs care, should I intervene? And what if the patient in need of care is in another country? I have wrestled with these dilemmas all my life: the need to make the right choice at the right time, and to live with the consequences. I've also faced up to making one of the biggest of choices: who to care for first?

*

A young family was moving into their new house in the hills surrounding the hospital. It was the week before Christmas and bitterly cold. While unpacking their belongings they momentarily lost sight of their toddler, who'd slipped out of the house and into the uncharted territory of the new garden. The excitement of the move gave way to the sheer panic of a lost child. The police were called and an officer, realising that what looked like a stone under the surface of a pond the parents didn't know was there was not what it seemed, jumped in and lifted the child's lifeless body to the surface. An ambulance raced through the streets until his still lifeless body was placed on the trolley before me. Children can survive immersion, particularly in cold water, for some time – but how long had the child been under? More than a few minutes but less than an hour was all we could ascertain. In any case, resuscitation had been commenced by a police officer, continued by the ambulance crew, and so would be completed by me. That's the way it is. If you wait to consider the whys and wherefores before proceeding, the delay will ensure the catastrophic brain damage you fear has now become a certainty. I placed a tube into the child's windpipe and oxygen into their lungs. I put drugs into their tiny veins while colleagues massaged the chest until, remarkably, their little heart began to beat again. But still they weren't breathing, and their eyes remained closed. A full team stood around the trolley on which the child's body looked so small, pondering how on earth we could get them safely through ten miles of Christmas traffic to the nearest paediatric intensive care unit. Every time we'd tried to move them, the child's heart rate became dangerously slow.

The journey would have to be smooth and regular, neither too quick nor too slow, and without any sudden braking or turns. A straight line without stopping. And then a voice at the back spoke up. The police officer who'd brought them from the water had never left their side. He had stood in his freezing wet clothes on the edge of the resuscitation room watching in silence for the three or four hours it had taken to get us to this point. 'The traffic won't be a problem,' he said, in a way that had no element of doubt or discussion disguised in its delivery. 'Give me half an hour.' It took that time to ready the child for the journey, connecting all the lines and slowly manoeuvring them into the ambulance. And then it started. We knew something strange was occurring as soon as we left the hospital. A posse of police motorcycle outriders surrounded the ambulance, each with its blue lights flashing. As we set off, they took it in turns to race ahead and clear the way, and as we passed a junction they were holding, to tuck in behind as their colleagues took their turn to race ahead and clear the next. At each and every one of the dozens of major junctions we sped through, a police officer, holding traffic to a standstill in all directions until we'd passed, raised their hand and saluted.

Why do I think of this so much after all these years? The child never fully recovered and later died, in spite of all our efforts and those of their wonderful parents. Not until some months later; but at least they died after we had done everything we could, I tell myself. The world they left had been lifted, if even only a little, by the coming together of so much human endeavour and spirit. Each of those police officers gave more than their job required: they gave something of themselves to a little child they didn't know and couldn't see behind the blacked-out windows of the ambulance as it passed. It still catches my breath when I see in my mind's eye that first police officer, standing in the dark, rain running down his face, and with his arms outstretched to stop the traffic, lifting his right hand further in a gesture of salute. I feel again the near bursting of my heart as this gesture was repeated time after time after time as we sped through the dark cold rainy night of winter.

But is this enough? Is it of itself, right? Should the drive to do good in the moment, borne high on an outpouring of emotion, override all that might follow? Amidst the cynicism and indifference I have seen people show, I have also seen an immense capacity to care. Surely success or failure is not only measured by outcome but also by the process? By the motives and values of those who do? But what about outcome, and the motives and values of those to whom good things are done? What about the cost of 'doing good?' I learned later that this child had been profoundly disabled by the lack of oxygen to their brain while under the water, requiring constant care and round the clock attention from devoted parents, before ultimately dying anyway. A philosopher might say I took a 'deontological' or 'virtuous' approach; that I did what I thought a good person would do.[4] Others might take the opposite view, a 'utilitarian' or 'consequentialist' approach, and calculate that the sum cost of resuscitation and prolonged treatment – in economic, social and emotional terms – outweighed the benefits of the child's short, and maybe painful, survival.[5] This dichotomy played out in the comments of my hospital colleagues. Some were supportive; others harshly critical. Each view was expressed to my face, just as they would be again when I started overseas aid work. This is a conflict that runs through all of medicine and plays out on a larger scale in the response to humanitarian emergencies. That human suffering must be addressed wherever it is found is the first human-itarian principle and is also commanded by much religious teaching.[6] The goodness, the benefit, lies mostly in the doing, it seems to me, irrespective of the outcome. But what about the outcome? Does the act actually do any good, or even result in harm? Doing nothing is neither neutral nor itself without conse-quence. To paraphrase author Mary B. Anderson, because 'doing' can do harm, it's a logical and moral fallacy to assume that 'not doing' – doing nothing – can do no harm.[7]

I saw early on in my treatment of another patient just how harm-ful doing nothing can be, and why we can't know the outcome – at least until it's over. I felt the lure of the saviour complex: the urge to step in in where I didn't necessarily belong, when it wasn't my patient.

*

I was on call for the intensive care unit, but it was an otherwise quiet weekend when I took a call from a senior nurse at the neighbouring maternity hospital. 'Please come over and look at a new mum,' she said. She looks really sick. 'What do her doctors think?' I asked. 'That's the problem,' she replied. 'They think she's not that ill, but I don't. Just come and see for yourself and see if you agree.' The correct thing to do would be for her doctors to refer the patient to me, but the nurse was sure that if I spoke first to her doctors, they would not agree to me seeing her. In fact, they'd already declined. There was something in the absence of any hubris in what she said – the obvious concern she had for her young patient and the cour-age she'd shown in the risk she'd taken in going over the heads of her own medical team – that meant I couldn't, and I believed shouldn't, ignore her. So, breaking all the rules, I went.

I arrived on the ward to find a very ill patient, a nervous midwife, and an angry doctor. I hadn't expected the doctor to be there, but the midwife had reflected and thought it best to tell him, reassured by knowing that I was now already on my way. I managed to persuade him that as I was here now we could see the patient together. It was immediately clear to me that she was developing sepsis and rapidly going downhill. Even her doctor now acknowledged that she was sicker than he first thought, and hesitantly agreed to let me take over her care. I knew we had to move quickly. I began her treatment immediately and arranged for an urgent transfer to the intensive care unit. As her midwife knew, and had anticipated, with sepsis, deterioration can be rapid, and too often unstoppable. She soon required artificial ventilation to keep her blood oxygen up and drugs to maintain her blood pressure. But to no avail; still she worsened. Her kidneys failed so we hooked her to a dialysis machine. When her urine flow stopped completely and there was no flicker of improvement anywhere to be seen, my senior colleagues began to talk of an inevitable, ghastly outcome. I spoke to her husband and prepared him for the worst: that he would take home his baby, but not her mother – his wife.

But she was so young and had a new baby. I would not give up on her – on them both. And then her heart slowed down. So slow now that she couldn't live very long if it didn't improve. Drugs didn't help. An unusual effect of the infection was slowing the 'conduction' of each beat through the heart – the electrical signals conveying the impulse. I suggested we fit a pacemaker. Apart from the risks of infection to her heart of this procedure, it was felt now by (almost) everyone that at this stage it would be futile: she was so ill, with all her organs failing, she seemed to be irretrievable and her death inevitable. But this view was not shared by everyone. Not by a senior charge nurse, who backed me, and although there was no wider enthusiasm, there were no outright objections either.

Luckily for her, the intensive care unit was not too busy. My other patients were stable or clearly recovering and there were no new admissions. So, in between caring for the others, I stationed myself at her bedside, ready to intervene, and carefully adjusted all of the machines and instruments in response to even the smallest changes in her condition. She was still no better. But no worse either. I snatched what sleep I could, sat up in a chair I placed by her bed, ready to intervene immediately if anything changed. Early one morning, the charge nurse who had come back on to start his day shift, gently shook me from my half sleep and, leaning over me smiling, pointed at the urine bag hanging below the side of the bed. There was clear urine dripping out of the tube, slowly but definitely. Her kidneys were beginning to work. She was still desperately ill, but by the middle of the day her heart was beating normally, and without the aid of the pacemaker. But when to remove it? The longer it was in, the greater the risk of infection to the heart, but with it present she was also protected. By the afternoon she was now clearly improving, and I removed the pacemaker. Her heart remained steady and her kidneys kept working.

She was still sedated and on a ventilator. Over the course of the next day I gradually reduced the drugs that were supporting her blood pressure, again without ill effect. The question now was when to try and wake her? The mood in the unit was brighter now, and those once dismissive of our efforts and her chances shared our new anxieties about if she would ever wake. If she did, what would she wake to? What disabilities, what suffering, had my heroics cemented into her future? We stopped the syringe drivers that pumped the drugs and waited. It was her fingers that moved first.

Then her eyelids. 'Open your eyes,' I said. And she did.

I gradually weaned her off the ventilator, and although still ill and very weak, she was out of immediate danger. I spoke again to her husband and gave him the cautiously optimistic news. Your job when dealing with relatives in these circumstances is to treat their hopes as a helium balloon: one that they hold and want to let go to see it rise, while you grab the string and keep tugging it down. Things can and do turn rapidly for the worse, and better that they stay ready for the killer blow than fall to a sucker punch. I always smile knowingly when doctors are reported as saying someone would never walk again, speak again, live again, and were shown to be wrong. I know their doctors were simply pulling down on the string of the helium balloon.

Tired, but not yet emotional, I handed over to my colleague as he came on duty. I watched him read through her notes and, placing them on the desk, he turned to me and said, 'Well done, but I wouldn't have done it. I wouldn't have gone to that hospital on the invitation of a nurse and without a formal referral from her consultant. I wouldn't have slept in the chair by her bed.' It wasn't said in praise but as fact. It had worked out in this case, but had I tried and risked too much? She made a full recovery, remembered little of the drama, and went home to her husband and her baby, now safely in her arms.

There is always risk in medicine, usually to the patient. But there can also be risk in delivering the care required of a good doctor. To the reputation of the doctor if things do not go as hoped for; to the health of the doctor when they do not know when or how to say enough is enough. And as I was to learn in the work I was to do later, for doctors in leadership positions, there are risks not only to themselves but to the welfare and even the lives of others who are also under their care: the members of their team. It is easier to lead others to where they already want to go and harder for them to follow you to where their instincts (and families) are telling them they don't. So how much do you persuade them to suppress their rational fears, and how much reassurance do you give them in order for them to join you? You are balancing your appetite for risk against theirs. You shouldn't choose for them, but your actions, in the moment, might mean that you do.

*

We left the last checkpoint in Iran before the border with Iraq and began our journey. It was 1991 and we were on our way to help Kurdish refugees fleeing Saddam and the aftermath of the first Gulf War. The thin tarmac layer gave way to dirt and the track got narrower. As we looked down the precipitous sides of the valleys, thin riverine snakes meandered far below. And still we climbed. When it seemed we could climb no further we drove up and down over mountaintops until we saw the scatterings of objects draped across distant peaks. These objects grew into tents as we drew closer. Thousands of people were camped precariously high in the clouds, thousands of feet up.

It was evening when our small convoy pulled into the centre of the camp. A mass of angry looking people thronged around our vehicles. Our interpreter was clearly frightened and said he thought it wasn't safe. They told us they had many sick and dying but no medicines. An Iranian government 'doctor' – we learned later he was a medical student – had for a while come once every few days to run a clinic from a small tent, but he had not been for some time. They knew the tent still held medicines, but it was roped shut and they dared not force it open. The camp was heavily guarded by

Iranian soldiers who would exercise discipline in the camp by periodically machine gunning over their heads from their post above. I
told the team to stay in the vehicle while I talked with the head of
the camp. He catalogued their many difficulties but emphasised the
closure of their clinic. Our interpreter, provided by the Iranian
Government and to all intents and purposes our minder, was now
very nervous indeed and told me to get back onto the truck. We
were to go back to Tehran, he said. It was too unstable. But I had
not come all this way to turn back now. In a moment of bravado, I
pushed my way through the crowds and stood before the medicine
tent. Flourishing my Swiss Army knife, I cut through the cords
binding the tent flaps closed and, throwing it wide open, turned to
the crowd and shouted, 'This clinic is now open!' The crowd
erupted in whistles and cheers, jumping up and down, punching
the air with their fists. The incomprehensibility of my English had
been instantly translated by the gesture and the sight of the gaping
tent flaps. My back was slapped, the team was pulled from their
vehicles in celebration, but I instantly thought 'now what?' As did
the Iranian Official. Thoughts that should perhaps have preceded
my cinematographic moment: a gesture, performed without
consultation with my colleagues. But things happen quickly and
the trade-off between making a safe retreat from a hostile crowd
and committing us to their mercy was not one that could be debated
at length, if at all. I'd made a decision and now we had to make it
work.

If the mood of the crowd was not to turn nasty again, we had to
hit the ground running. I instructed the team to unload and make
ready to set to work immediately. As my eyes adjusted to the scene
before me, I realised that a queue, of women mainly, had already
been waiting by the medicine tent. Waiting for days, in fact, for the

Iranian doctor who never came. And the first three women in the queue were holding babies. I took a closer look. The women were sat cross-legged on the ground, cradling their infants in their laps, shielding them with their veils. As they each drew back this curtain, the picture of a very sorry, very sick child, rigid with end-stage meningitis, was revealed. So rigid were they now, their spines were arched and their heads held back in the classic picture of opisthotonos, now so rarely seen in the west.[8] The temporary euphoria following my grand opening of the tent evaporated in an instant. My heart sank. I felt sick. Sick for the anguish of these parents who faced the inevitable death of their babies, now too ill to respond to treatment. Sick too for having raised false hopes in these poor suffering people, but sick too with just more than a little fear that as they and others like them died, our position high on this lonely mountain, far from contact with the outside world, might just become even more hazardous.

I rallied the team and asked them to start work on the babies. I knew the position was hopeless, but we had to at least do something. The look in their eyes mirrored these feelings and they whisked the infants into their arms and established intravenous (IV) lines. We agreed they obviously had meningitis but what type was impossible to tell. We therefore decided to treat them with simple broad-spectrum antibiotics intravenously and to rehydrate them with drips. With the treatment regimes established and a nurse constantly by their sides, we set about organising our mission.

We quickly established a basic treatment tent and commandeered the tent next door as an 'intensive care unit' for those who were more seriously ill. That first night was long and hard. Early the next morning I looked in on the three infants, expecting only the worst. The mattresses where I had last seen them prostrate were now bare and their places in the tent taken by three other infants, sat on their mother's knees eating breakfast. I looked in sorrow to the nurse who had been there all through the night. She was smiling. The mothers were smiling. I was confused. I looked at the three new infants and saw now they had IV lines in their little arms. I thought too I recognised their faces. As I dared to believe in miracles, the tears that welled in the nurse's eyes and the look of weary peace on the faces of their mothers told me that a miracle had indeed occurred. Still very ill, but clearly now destined to live, these were indeed the very same children I'd seen the night before. I went out into the sunlight and looked around the camp. The days were getting warmer and there was lots of work to be done. I was not to know it then, but despite snakebites, typhoid and mine strikes, no infant, child or adult would die under our care.

I have never forgotten these children. I have never forgotten how far a tiny drop of medicine can spread in a pool of need. I have also heard the medical head of an international children's charity, now retired, warn publicly of the dangers of emergency medical aid to 'developing' countries, fearing that mothers might learn to expect their children to live and so suffer more when they die. Such sentiments are aired only as an excuse: as an excuse for tolerating such terrible differentials in health care across this small world of ours; as an excuse for agencies doing the easier things, like counting the dead, instead of treating the living.

Day by day the camp became more organised. Water that was shipped in every day by huge great tankers became more plentiful and food was not only distributed more frequently, but also sold in small wayside markets.

But still the patients kept on coming. We were told the camp to which we ministered was 20,000 strong. As news of our presence

spread it became clear that patients were trekking across the mountaintops from other camps, carrying their sick and their wounded.
The work was never ending. One afternoon a colleague asked me
what to make of a case he'd just admitted. The fever, the rash all
suggested typhoid. We consulted the textbooks we always carried
with us and searched our memories and experiences. Yes, it was
typhoid. And over the next few days more cases followed. But each
responded well to treatment and there were no fatalities. We also
saw malaria in the camp, imported as a keepsake from Iraq. Amongst
the most tragic cases were the children who were burned as a
secondary consequence of that scourge of modern warfare: landmines. Both sides had laid landmines. They were everywhere, but
we couldn't be more specific than that. Days were punctuated by
the explosive thud of a mine strike, usually blowing to bits the
family goat or cow. Each explosion brought a rush to see that it
really was an animal and not a child, but confirmation brought only
some relief as the loss of milk or meat heralded only a new set of
problems.

There was, of course, no electricity to the camp, so cooking was
done over open fires, and oil lamps lit the insides of the tents. The
dangers of burning lamps and open fires in such confined spaces was
magnified horribly by the inability of children to run around freely
and play. The area on which the camp was built had been a battle-
field for the long and bloody Iran–Iraq War and had changed hands
several times. Children had to play indoors and when their games of
chase ended in collision with an oil lamp, the tent caught fire. We did
our very best for these scarred and wounded children, but their faces
would forever tell the story of their childhood on the run.

At night the Kurdish PKK would bring their wounded.[9] These
fighters filed silently but not unnoticed into the respectful reception

of the camp. During the day Iranian guards would push their way to the front of any queue and demand we give attention to their minor aches and pains. There was always a constant tension building and abating between the camp, the guards and ourselves. It was important for the guards to see us as impartial and the camp to know we were not uncaring. So, we always made the guards wait, but gave them some attention. After a while, the guards began to be more aggressive and would arrive at our sleeping quarters, availing themselves of what we were cooking. They eyed our possessions and brooded in silence. On most occasions we confounded their threatening behaviour with a pre-emptive invitation to share the meal, even before they helped themselves.

One day the camp was visited from above. A helicopter landed without warning on a terrace just above our row of tents. I was working lower down in the treatment tent at the time and looked up in horror as the down draft from the rotor blades raised a massive swirling cloud of dust, our tents straining to pull away from their moorings. A body went hurtling over the side to the terrace below. We all ran to where we saw her fall. It was one of our senior female nurses who had been injured. She had badly contused her shoulder joint and was out of action for much of the remainder of the mission. When the pain became more bearable, she insisted on taking over much of the running of the camp, but her injury was a reminder to us all of the vulnerability of our isolation and just how quickly things could turn. It brought home to me the risks I was encouraging others to take.

Whenever people are in fear, it has been my experience that they have the uncanny knack of inventing stories to make life just that little bit worse. It had happened previously in Armenia and it happened again here in Iran. A popular rumour for a while was that the Iranians were going to bomb the camp, in the same way that tales of Russians bombing Leninakan (now Gyumri) had taken hold when we were in Armenia a few years previously. I began to have my own doubts when fighter jets sortied overhead and the day we watched in awe as a cruise missile graced across the sky, I almost became a believer. There did reach a point where we all feared greatly for our safety and after the cruise missile had first mesmerised then terrified us, these feelings reached a peak. Some team members preferred not to sleep and stayed awake watching for whatever might befall us. I remember that on that evening when fear was at its greatest, feeling so very tired after a particularly arduous clinical shift, that I lay in my tent and thought only of sleep. If they bomb me in the night, I remember thinking, so what? I experienced a similar feeling some years later at the height of the war in Sarajevo. NATO bombing appeared imminent and Serb retaliation possibly only hours away. There was nothing I could do then. Escape was impossible, so I slept. And as I would do in Bosnia, I awoke fresh the next day and the fears of imminent attack retreated.

Work carried on as usual until the arrival of the International Red Cross. We had been wondering for some time how we could ever leave. The work just kept on coming. But they had heard of our work and found us. We talked about cases and they confirmed the presence of typhoid and malaria in other camps. They seemed genuinely impressed with what we had achieved and discussed a phased handover to their care. The first thing they did in the coming days was to deliver a brand new, purpose built large hospital facility. The day we carried our patients, babies in our arms, drips held high in the air, in procession to this new facility was indeed a day to remember. It marked a turning point. The camp had food and water and a permanent adequate medical facility. The Red Cross would soon be sending a doctor and nurse who could stay on much longer. The health of the camp was stable; it was only maintenance and not emergency care that was now required. It was time to be thinking of going home.

But how to get home? In the year between this and our first mission to Iran in response to a large earthquake, things had opened up enough for a weekly Swissair flight to be added to the Iranair flights we knew. The demand for flights was so great however, and the corruption at the airport so rife, that securing a booking for a large group of foreigners was going to prove problematic. It would likely take days or even weeks of wrangling in Tehran, so estimating time of arrival in the UK and a return to our usual tasks was going to prove difficult. It was then that I thought of seeking the help of the Iranian captain in charge of guarding the camp. I knew he had a field telephone and wondered if he had any means of wider contact. 'I am sorry, my friend,' he said whimsically to our translator. 'I only have this military phone that connects with my superiors in Tehran.' 'But there are telephone wires that run nearby,' I replied. I had seen them. 'Oh yes,' he said with a smile, 'but they do not stop here. The only way to use them would be to illegally break into their circuit.' His smile grew wider. 'I need to speak with my colleagues in Manchester,' I said. As ever, these words when uttered abroad, provoked a response of 'Ah, Manchester United, Bobby Charlton!' I gave him the number of our travel agent in Manchester. Eventually a young soldier was ordered up the telegraph pole and a handset placed in my hand. The man at the top of the pole spoke to Tehran who connected us through to the UK. As if booking my annual holiday, I stood in the open by a telegraph pole on a mountain in Iran and asked the travel agent to do all that they could to reserve us our seats. That was it.

Choices

The call ended, we packed up our things, said our goodbyes and began the two-day journey back to Tehran.

Our problems were not quite over when we got to the airport itself. We'd made it in time for the weekly flight but only just, and time was ticking away. The Swissair desk was so tantalisingly close, easily seen beyond the customs desk, the Swissair man I had been told to look out for was to my amazement and relief there waving to me. But the customs officer was not friendly. He saw me waving and our hurry and slowed everything down to a crawl. Ahead of us in the queue, a diplomat had already been relieved of a Persian carpet, illegally hidden in his baggage. The official wanted more. When it was our turn, he eyed us up and down and narrowed his eyes on the mountain of boxes that accompanied our place in the queue. Walking along the line we made, he stopped at a nurse and without a word began to rifle through her shoulder bag. He took a chocolate bar she had been saving from the bag and provocatively peeled back the wrapper and chewed it slowly in her face, deliberately inviting protest. She looked at me and my expression said 'Leave it. Say nothing. We're almost home.' He followed her gaze to me and in English barked 'Where are your papers?' I showed him all that I had, including an inventory of all our equipment and the import licence for the medical goods. We'd been told that even if the goods were being brought into the country to aid our humanitarian mission, we would still need to pay for an import licence. I thought we had all the bases covered. 'But where are your export licences?' he asked slyly. I hadn't seen that one coming. Now here was a quandary. If I said we hadn't got them he was more than likely to deny or certainly delay our exit, and we'd certainly miss the plane and it would be at least a week before we might get enough places on another. Best case scenario. Worst case, we might have been imprisoned for attempting to smuggle medical goods out of the country. 'Every piece of medical equipment that leaves must have a licence.' he said. 'Well that's lucky,' I replied, 'because all the equipment you see listed on the import licence has been donated and the boxes before you contain only camping equipment.' He insisted on taking a look. Not unreasonable in retrospect, I suppose – I was lying. It's true that at the end of a mission we did donate all the consumables, drugs bandages etc., but certain specialised pieces of surgical instrumentation were part of our core team equipment, and they always travelled back with us. I hadn't a clue which of the dozen or so boxes of equipment before us they were scattered amongst. But nor did he. Was he going to make us dismantle the pile and open every one? He might well do. If he did so we'd miss the plane anyway. But the queue behind was now larger than ever and he was under mounting pressure to get things moving again. He chose a box slap bang in the middle. We had to dismantle the stack quickly and remove the seals and stand back in silence as he opened its lid. 'Camping equipment?' he said softly. My heart stopped. With a look of total disappointment, he pulled a tent from its depths and angrily told us to get a move on. He turned his attentions to the next victims in the queue and we boarded the plane with only minutes to spare.

The circumstances that had prompted our mission to Kurdistan were very grave and the suffering of this people continues till today. But we did what we could when we could, and left with a tangible sorrow for their plight, tempered by the feeling of a difficult job well done.

*

Choices

Only twelve months before, in 1990, I was also in Iran, but then without a visa, without an embassy to turn to, and in the basement of an Iranian military hospital. 'These are the patients you must treat first.' said General Moshiri, the head of the hospital. A few days earlier, just after midnight on 21 June 1990, a very powerful earthquake of 7.4 magnitude had violently shaken the Manjil–Rudbar area north west of Tehran. When the counting was over, and the bodies retrieved or otherwise, up to 50,000 Iranians were found to have died and more than 100,000 of the survivors had been injured. A dozen or so of the most seriously injured lay in a row before me, each on an old metal-framed hospital bed and covered in a stained, crumpled blanket. The General's chosen four were all older men: each unresponsive and all breathing slowly and shallowly. The catheters emerging from under their blankets were clear and snaking into empty collection bags. Their legs, exposed by turning back the blankets, were black, smelly, and visibly bubbling with obvious gas gangrene. Turning my gaze a little to the right, I saw a young woman: semi-conscious, toxic and with one leg black below the knee. She was breathing relatively well, and her catheter was yellow with urine: its collection bag one third full. Next to her was a young man similarly injured but perhaps a little more alert. The remaining queue was a similar mix of men and women, mostly young, and all with at least something in their catheter bag. I looked to my team of UK doctors and nurses, each of whom had volunteered to respond with me to a request for help from the Iranian Red Crescent Society. Our experience told us that all the patients needed their crushed and infected limbs removed immediately if they were to have any chance of survival. The first four were likely to die anyway, I felt, whereas the young woman was on the cusp. If the mangled limb was removed now, she might survive. The man next to her would also more likely survive with immediate surgery; the others, though ill, could wait a short while.

We discussed this amongst ourselves with General Moshiri looking on, and agreed that his favoured four would almost inevitably die, even if treated in the best UK facility. They were clearly septic, unresponsive, barely breathing, and in kidney failure. We had limited operating capacity and we reasoned that taking the young man and woman first was likely to be the most effective course of action. They at least had a reasonable chance of survival with surgery, and none without. 'So, we are agreed?' I asked the team. 'We take the young woman and the young man first?' I remember them saying: 'It's your decision.' Such are the burdens of leadership.

I explained my views to the General, who protested that his chosen patients were the most ill and so needed our western expertise more than the others. At the same time, he expressed his doubts about the use of amputation, particularly in young women, and in the volatile environment in which we, as foreigners, found ourselves. I explained our reasoning and recognised in his demeanour that he was not in fundamental disagreement. He managed to imply, despite hostile onlookers, that decisions, choices, made by transient foreigners bore fewer consequences than those made by those, like him, required to stay and live with such consequences. He neither agreed nor objected, but acquiesced, and we took our chosen patients to the operating theatre. All went well and they clearly improved. On returning to the ward, the first two beds had been stripped following the death of their occupants, and the second two contained patients now even closer to death. In sight, but out of earshot, the General and his colleagues were speaking to the distraught relatives of those we'd left behind.

Choices

I can still doubt my decision, despite all the evidence that says that I was right. I have told and retold this story in countless lectures and tutorials, and each time I wait for the hand to go up and a voice to say, 'but you could have …' There is so much a part of me that knows I did the right thing, made the right choice, and still a part of me that feels so heavily for the ones that we passed over: the ones we chose to leave to die.

The issue before us was that we did not have the capacity to give the best treatment to them all, all at once; we would have to choose who would be first. No patient had a guaranteed chance of survival with or without surgery, but the sooner the source of the infection that was triggering their sepsis and kidney failure (the leg) was removed, the greater would be their chance of survival. Conversely, the longer each waited for surgery, the greater would be their risk of dying or deteriorating to a level that would render them beyond help. To resolve it we looked to triage to maximize the number of survivors and do the greatest good for the greatest number. We adhered to the notion that the moral right or wrong of an action is determined solely by its consequences, as opposed to things being right or wrong regardless of their consequences. And as the architect of triage, Baron Dominique-Jean Larrey himself had advocated, 'those who are dangerously wounded should receive the first attention, without regard to rank or distinction,' we chose our patients according to the urgency of their condition rather than their rank – mindful that we were in Tehran, where men outranked women, and older men outranked younger men. Larrey had also recognised 'how quickly the wounded are victimised by tetanus and sepsis, and how their condition rapidly improved after amputation': an observation of particular relevance to the clinical presentation of the patients we saw in Tehran.

*

It was June 1990 when a fierce earthquake had shaken the north-west region of Iran centred on the town of Rasht. Since responding to an earthquake in Armenia two years previously I had met and talked with many individuals and agencies involved in the international aid scene and our medical team was now registered with the United Nations Disaster Relief Organisation (UNDRO). It was they who forwarded a request for the services of our team in Iran to the Overseas Development Administration, who met the costs of our mission to a country with no British Embassy, no diplomatic relations with the UK, and with no visas. We needn't have worried. Visas were issued on arrival and we were taken to a nice hotel. It may have flourished a large flag in the foyer saying 'Down with America' but otherwise we felt safe and well looked after. When dawn broke we were taken by coach to begin our work in the Iranian Air Force Military Hospital, Tehran.

The hospital was full to overflowing with injured men, women, and children. Obviously in great pain and each with a story of loss and bereavement. But each with an air of stoicism and acceptance. My words of sympathy for their terrible loss were dismissed in an instant. 'It is our loss,' I was told. 'Don't add to it with your miserable faces and your words of sorrow. You have come to help and that it is good. So, help and we will recover.' I felt like my face had been slapped. But it worked. I put away my cloak of foreign sympathy and just set to work. I smiled, and my patients smiled back.

Working under the strict regime of the Mullahs was not as restrictive as we had feared it might be. True, when one of the team foolishly took a picture of the now defunct US embassy, his camera was mysteriously stolen later that day; but the authorities did apologise and provide an 'identical replacement', now devoid of the original film. While we were given what appeared superficially to be a degree of freedom, we were accompanied everywhere by our 'interpreter', just as we would be the following year in Kurdistan, and were never allowed to leave the hotel in the evenings or the hospital in the day. Our equipment was held in the hospital, guarded day and night by armed soldiers. One afternoon, somewhat fatigued by the feeling of imprisonment, benign as it might have been, a nurse and I combined rebellion with a shared childhood experience. As we were searching through our boxes of drugs and dressings, I got to chatting about how all this seemed a long way away from Manchester. It turned out we had both survived Irish Catholic upbringings and what's more we had both been to Irish dancing lessons. Kicking your legs high with your back straight as a poker were common sufferings and the slip jig a shared ambition. As we reminisced and giggled about the arcane rituals presided over by those tyrannical mistresses of the dance our parents said were teachers, the young revolutionary guards looked on, with disapproval. 'What the hell,' I thought. We ducked out of sight behind a pillar and knotted our arms behind us to form a figure of eight. For perhaps the first time, an eight-hand reel was to be performed in post-revolutionary Tehran. One, two, three, four, I beat out the time. And, humming 'The Irish Washerwoman', we emerged locked together, sweeping through their field of vision. There followed silence. Absolute silence. In for a penny, we thought, and re-entered from the wings to pass once again before their staring eyes, jaws on the floor, and AK-47 rifles about to fall from their hands. On regaining safety behind the pillar, we simply set about our usual business. No more was said.

We did go to the scene of the earthquake, but only after weeks of work in the hospital. Help was needed to review all those patients not injured enough to have required transfer to Tehran, but nevertheless still in need of care. It was a stunning journey overland to the edge of the Caspian Sea and for a while we forgot the purpose of our journey. But when the sickly-sweet smell of death filtered through our nostrils, we knew exactly why we were there and what we had to do. The villagers were resilient and accepting and doing everything they could to restore their shattered lives. Treatment was simple and effective – changing dressings, giving supplies of painkillers and antibiotics. Viewing the scene put our work in Tehran into perspective. We knew now that all those who had needed immediate medical care had received it. It was time to go home.

3.

The Hardest Month

Armenia / Lockerbie

Early December 1988. Mikhail Gorbachev, the President of what was then the Soviet Union, was visiting the USA. Bitter enemies of the Cold War appeared to be reaching out to each other, and Gorbachev was greeted in New York with the classic 'ticker tape' parade. Almost at the same time it seemed to me then, a huge earthquake struck Armenia – a Soviet Republic in the south of the country – and the joy and optimism that surrounded the visit was instantly clouded in a terrible sadness. Not since the Second World War had the world looked to the Soviet Union and offered to help; not since the War had the Soviet Union indicated it might accept. The Press Association ran a story about the call-out for trauma specialists. It was read by a journalist at the Manchester Evening News who had recently covered the activities of the South Manchester Accident Rescue Team (SMART). She rang the hospital, I answered the phone, my fate was sealed. She asked me why 'the SMART team' was not going to the earthquake in Armenia. 'Because nobody's asked,' I replied. Not flippantly, just reactively. One of the team members had already suggested to me that we offer our services, but I had pushed back saying we hadn't been asked so we should wait. After all, there must be others better equipped and experienced to respond to such a large-scale disaster, not least the Soviet Union themselves, I reasoned. And who would fund it?

But that phone call and my response triggered a chain of events that ultimately led to me sitting in a BBC Radio studio in Manchester while Chris Patten, the then Minister for Overseas Development, sat in the 'Today' studio for BBC Radio 4 in London. The issue for On Air 'discussion' was essentially that the Soviets said they needed trauma teams; we had a trauma team; the government was sending aid to Armenia, but not trauma teams. They were sending tents and blankets in line with their usual response, but not personnel. At the time there was a prevailing ethos that emergency aid had little impact and real change came from developmental aid. Some years later, a very senior civil servant within the ODA was to tell me during his visit to Sarajevo where I was working, that he didn't 'believe' in emergency medical aid. I hadn't regarded it as a matter of faith. This split between emergency humanitarian assistance and developmental aid persists still, though the dichotomy is not as great as evidence replaces simple belief.

'So why won't you fund the team?', Brian Redhead asked Chris Patten. To his disappointment and my relief (there would be no on air spat) he replied, 'Contact my office and we'll give you all the support you need'. And that was that. I phoned the ODA as instructed and after an initially muted response, it seemed all systems were now set to go. We assembled a team of experienced doctors and nurses, including specialists in the management of crush injuries (as specified by the Russians) and waited for the next instruction. Momentum was gathering and colleagues in Edinburgh were putting together a follow-up team should it be required. A third could be mobilised from across Manchester. Meanwhile we watched news reports of the growing death toll and the appalling weather conditions that were hampering rescue efforts. We were informed by ODA that a large amount of supplies and equipment had already been sent and we need only take ourselves. We were also told that protective clothing would not be required. I was not convinced and rang the appropriate government department for further assistance, explaining that I was going to Armenia as part of the British Aid effort, and could I have some environmental advice. 'Wrap up well, we've heard it's rather chilly,' was the reply. I was so stunned I wrote it down word for word. It was -20°C and falling on our first night. My image of a well-oiled government machine moving effortlessly into action began to crumble. Undeterred, I rang my brother who brought me all his spare chill room clothing from his meat depot and I took the team to a ski outfitter in Manchester.

We had understood that we would join other British rescue workers on an RAF Hercules and fly direct to the scene. This plan evaporated without explanation and as the death toll rose hour by hour, we waited over the weekend for the next available scheduled Aeroflot flight to Moscow. I have since recounted this and my feeling of consternation each time I have spoken publicly about my work. After a lecture in London I was pulled to one side by a man who introduced himself as a military officer. The Hercules was ready to take you all he said, but it was stood down on orders from above. How far above? I asked. He explained it was Mrs Thatcher's idea, to make the Russians pay.

This further delay weakened our chances of making any significant difference to the acutely injured, but we now felt obliged to see it through, gain from the experience, and be better prepared next time. Early on the Monday morning I kissed my three small children goodbye as they lay sleeping in their beds. It was my eldest daughter's tenth birthday. We arrived at Heathrow to be greeted with the news of the Clapham Junction rail crash. A major disaster at home while we were on our way to Moscow. The fear we were experiencing was joined by sadness and the echoes in our heads of what our critics might say about our choices.

As the plane took off, I found myself chatting to the British aid worker in the seat next to mine. He was a search and rescue firefighter. 'It'll be your first mission, then,' he said. 'How did you guess?', I replied. 'I didn't see you checking the hold of the plane to make sure all your kit got on board.' What did he mean? We'd checked it in. This was Heathrow. Why watch it go in the hold? How did you get to watch it go in the hold? I was to find out the answer to some of these questions in stages. The first stage was when we arrived in Moscow and none of our kit came off the plane. We only had the small amount we had taken on board as hand luggage. 'Not loaded' was the only reply we could get at the time. I got a more detailed reply on my return home. By persistence and the good offices of those who tried to help, I got my answer. The kit – medical and surgical supplies in great quantities – had been removed 'on the instructions of one of your team.' 'No way!' was my immediate reaction. 'True!' was the response. Only it wasn't my team. The airport authorities couldn't distinguish between the individual components of the 'British aid team'. When that search and rescue team arrived late at check-in, they were told there was no room in the hold for all their equipment. 'No worries,' they'd said. 'We'll tell you what you can take off.' The Firefighter sat next to me had told them to remove our kit and replace it with theirs, while the airport workers thought they were simply prioritising the kit of the overall team. The firefighter hadn't checked with me or anyone else in SMART and didn't tell me on the flight how blighted he'd now made our deployment. This was my first, but sadly not the last, example of competitive humanitarianism. To get your organisation seen to be there at all costs. To the battle of the stickers – getting your organisation's logo seen on camera at any price.

On arrival in Moscow we were received by British Embassy Officials. As leader of the team, I was briefed directly. Over a hundred Russian military rescue workers had already died in two separate plane crashes in the earthquake area as air traffic control had been lost. A chemical plant had been damaged, and the status of a nuclear reactor in the region was unknown. There was also a significant risk of major aftershocks. 'Our man in Moscow', stating he had our best interests at heart, recommended we simply stay in the city, 'where we can find plenty of good work for you to do' and return safely to the UK in a week or so to a British public who, he could assure me, would remain none the wiser. So much of what he said was shocking, but most shocking was his confidence that he could and would mislead the British public, and his confidence that we would be complicit. I could accept he might have genuine concerns for our safety, and some very real diplomatic worries about how to deal with a number of dead British doctors deep in the Soviet Union. But if so, he could have suggested we simply turned around and went home. But no, having arrived in the USSR the politics that delayed our departure now demanded we stay. Having just learned about competitive humanitarianism, I now learned about political humanitarianism. I was set to reject his offer out of hand but felt duty bound to offer it to the team. I have always been painfully aware of the complex pressures at play in 'volunteering'. It is not just you that is dicing with your future. When volunteering for dangerous missions you are risking the lives of all those who depend upon you for leadership. I never ask for reasons if people withdraw at any stage. I know what they are.

The team shared my response, and we left for Yerevan, the capital of Armenia. There were many rescue workers waiting for transport. We queued for aeroplanes, rather like waiting for a bus. And frighteningly like a bus, we just got on. No tickets, no seat numbers. The only criterion was that you could show you were a rescue worker. 'I'm with them,' said an unknown figure as we scrambled onto an ageing Russian aeroplane. True, he was with us, in that he had stood alongside us in the queue, but we had no idea who he was. We soon found out. As soon as the plane took off, he opened the large hold-all we'd assumed was medical or rescue kit and removed his large video camera. He was a freelance roving TV reporter who filmed the flight – filmed the piles of dead bodies, mayhem and misery – then moved off to the next telegenic disaster. But not before he'd latched onto one of the team and seduced him into breaking ranks and going with him in the night, alone, to be filmed in the rubble while I was searching for the coordination centre and the team were establishing a base. After hours of great anxiety, our team member re-joined us, and the cameraman moved on.

We were also accompanied on the flight by a member of the British Embassy in Moscow. Or so we were told. He was to be our minder – our fixer – and help us get around once in Armenia. He disembarked with us but I never saw him again. He was gone by the time we were leaving the airport. I heard of him though. Some months later *The Times* reported that he'd been expelled from the USSR for spying. This was still the Cold War, and the opportunity to get someone unchaperoned into a Soviet Republic, particularly one whose mind and watchful gaze were elsewhere, was too good an opportunity to miss. Even at the expense of helping fellow British citizens going into danger.

The airport at Yerevan was in chaos. Stacked by the runway I saw a pile of Thomas Splints. These are large metal frames used in the UK in the past for the treatment of fractures of the femur. But they weren't used in Armenia. The money that had paid for these well-meaning but useless gifts, that was burned in fuel flying their considerable weight across thousands of miles, was no longer available to purchase things they could have used. The space that had been available for the very things they might have used had been filled with things they could not. It is not a benign gesture to send things off to disasters. It has consequences. Time and again we send things where what is really needed is money. Regardless of whether the cost of their transport is greater than their worth. Regardless of whether the space they occupy in transport and storage reduces capacity for the essential. 'But you never really know where the money ends up,' I always hear. This is true to an extent, but giving to large reputable agencies guarantees some sort of security, as money can be more easily spent at the point of need and a paper trail examined. But if you send toys, clothes, and blankets, I know exactly where they will go. Usually nowhere, often into warehouses, and not uncommonly into the pockets of the corrupt. Sometimes they do get through, but too often at the expense of the needy. The biggest threat to emergency aid is a lack of co-ordination and co-operation. Let the big agencies decide what is needed and provide them with the money. It's for the best.

We were herded into a battered old coach and driven up the mountains to the city of Leninakan, the largest city to be struck by the earthquake. As we climbed higher, the temperature fell lower and lower, as did our spirits. Thousands of people were streaming

out of the earthquake zone and flooding towards us and around
our coach, like a flock of sheep around a farmer's Land Rover. We
were swimming slowly upstream against this human tide; the last
vehicle in a convoy of lorries snaking up a long, long road, and
each laden to overflowing with empty coffins. On reaching the
city, the scale of devastation was overwhelming. All my years of
work in A&E – the blood, the suffering, the tragedy – had not
prepared me for this: the scale was simply too great. The feeling
was that of drowning, being completely suffocated by death and
destruction. There was nowhere to look to avoid the horror of
crushed bodies, blood oozing out from between the collapsed
floors of buildings like jam from a sandwich. The sickly-sweet
smell of rotting corpses hung in the frozen air – an unnaturally
warm sensation in cold nostrils. It was growing dark and even
colder. I hurried through the unlit streets to where I was told the
Mayor was briefing rescue teams. Lamp posts had toppled and the
roads and pavements were rippled by the waves of the earthquake.
Cars had been abandoned or crashed during the tremor. In the
dark I tripped and fell through the open window of a car straddled
across the sidewalk. My head was now in the lap of a man, long
dead, his eyes and mouth wide open, frozen solid over the steering
wheel. Too shocked to scream, I squeezed myself out and ran and
eventually found the office of the Mayor, who directed our efforts
to where he thought there might still be survivors. We knew the
delay in leaving the UK meant we were unlikely to be of much use
in the early rescue phase, but we were ready to help in the hospitals. In any case, the majority of rescue and immediate aid is
provided to the victims of earthquakes by its survivors.
International help is often too late to make much of an impact on
the rescue, and always too late to significantly alter the immediate

death toll. However, the secondary death toll, people dying from lack of treatment, can be influenced by continuing assistance. The local doctors may need help so they can rest and be with their families or look for their own missing. The demands of the disaster leave little spare capacity for the everyday medical and surgical problems that don't stop just because of the earthquake. We saw that with our own eyes, and in our future deployments we broadened our remit to supporting the local practitioners in maintaining an essential emergency healthcare service and widened the skill mix of the team.

We did have some kit that we had hand-carried onto the aircraft, and certainly enough to be of assistance if the rescue workers should find anyone still alive at this relatively late stage. But they didn't. We made camp on a mountain top with some American paramedics and were ferried around the wrecked city by the Austrian Army. Canadian search and rescue dogs sniffed out corpses below the ones we ourselves could smell, and the night grew even colder. At night in the camp an Austrian military officer confirmed the threat of civil unrest and that a curfew had now been imposed. In the quiet of the night we heard the sporadic gunfire of its enforcement. Tensions were high. Heavy lifting gear flown in by the Austrians had been hijacked at gunpoint by local Armenians and Austrian rescue workers had been forced to rework a site by the relatives of those trapped inside. It was twelve hours before the rescue workers were released unharmed, having found no one alive in the rubble. Red Cross workers told me they had rescued someone only a few hours earlier: a pregnant woman. She had been trapped for several days under the rubble and had delivered her baby alone underground. Unable to move to cradle her new-born, she had held it between her legs all that time. The baby was now dead, and her legs too were lifeless. She was the last documented survivor. I was to meet this tragic woman less than twenty-four hours later working on the intensive care unit in Leninakan. Both her legs had been amputated, and although on a life support machine, she was clearly in the last few hours of her life. She died the next day.

Being at the top of a mountain far behind the iron curtain and in the immediate aftermath of an earthquake was troublesome in itself, but it was made worse by the rumour mill working within the foreign rescue workers. I was constantly told the Azerbaijanis were going to take rescue workers hostage. There was ongoing conflict between Armenia and Azerbaijan, as there still is today, which gave a small kernel of truth around which the rumours and lies could crystallise. The Russians were going to bomb the area to reduce the risk of epidemics, was one. There were in fact Russian jets flying overhead, and there was a profound fear of epidemics, as there often is after an earthquake – unjustified in practice. But the two were not connected. Nevertheless, rumours feed on fear and everyone was very afraid.

The light the new dawn threw on the day only made the picture darker. At each street corner the coffins were stacked in piles, some with lids askew, the clothes of their contents fluttering in the chill wind. Body collection trucks circled the city, removing the coffins like a macabre refuse truck collecting bins outside a house. They were taken to a sports stadium where they lay silently waiting for the heartbroken to stream in and stake their claims. The threat of civil unrest and the recent civil conflict lent an additional air of tension, and tanks rolled down the streets where people wandered. Troops fired over the heads of those too impatient (or hungry) to wait their turn in a bread queue. When I spoke about these experiences later, in a public meeting, a member of the audience stood up and rather aggressively denied that there had ever been Russian tanks on the streets. I was unclear why he was saying this and who he was representing. When the meeting was finished I was approached by an American who told me not to worry about the 'tank denier'; he was in the US military and they had been tracking my every move by satellite. He agreed that tanks were rolling by while we were trying to listen to the noises of the trapped. My first thought was 'why didn't he say so publicly in the meeting?' But I knew why.

A sleepless night of ultimately futile but constant effort convinced us to go where we now knew we should have been – in the main hospitals. The survivors, of course, want you to stay by the wreckage of their houses as a symbol that there is still some lingering hope. They will not give up. Rescue workers would mark a building after it had been searched. When they moved on to the next, the family of those trapped inside would wipe it off and tell the next group of passing rescue workers that the building was yet to be explored. A crane driver was held at gunpoint when he tried to move to the next pile of rubble.

A military plane transported us back to Yerevan where more meetings with officials led us to the intensive care unit and wards of the main hospital. We split into pairs and did what we could, where we could. The local doctors were exhausted and pleased to share their burden.

When we later returned home, we found that great play was made by the international media of the apparent chaos that surrounded the rescue effort, with little reference to the enormous difficulties of scale that faced the authorities. The official death toll was 25,000. But that was 25,000 bodies, or at least apparently matching body parts, found, put in a box, formally identified, and the paperwork completed. The true death toll was much greater. Moreover, the earthquake was at the top of a mountain, in sub-zero temperatures, on the edge of a country so large that its administrative centre was as far away from the epicentre as London is from Algiers. But the actions of journalists in this regard only echoed similarly repeated misconceptions that often surround the reporting of large-scale emergencies, and disasters in general. The most enduring falsehood retold again and again after each major 'natural' disaster is that the unburied dead pose a threat to the living. This is simply not so. Dead bodies harbour no more and no less infection than they did the moment before they died. Being dead does not create infection; it can only allow the release of what's already there. And dead bodies don't move. Any infection stays where it is. Living people, on the other hand, do move around and it is they that are far more likely to spread infection, particularly when there is a lack of sanitation. But if you die of an infection that can live on in bodily fluids for some time after death, then dead bodies are a risk: ebola and cholera are two examples. But the victims of earthquakes did not die from an infection. They died from their injuries. Concerns reported about large numbers of bodies contaminating the water table with faecal matter have been shown to be unfounded. Most of the millions of bodies buried in the United Kingdom are now inevitably below the water table. It is the faeces of the earthquake survivors contaminating their hands unwashed for lack of water that is a more immediate threat to their health and the overcrowded conditions in temporary camps that in practice causes disease outbreak. I understand the distress, fear and even revulsion provoked by living alongside the unburied dead, but this will be less than the permanent heartache and misery caused by their loved ones disappearing forever into mass graves, hastily dug and filled in response to unfounded fears.

The emergency phase drew quickly to a close and team members were increasingly anxious to get back to the UK once their highly specialised skills were no longer required there in Armenia. While most of us could have stayed a bit longer, the team member who had gone off with the cameraman revealed he had made only limited back up plans for being away and really needed to get back. Rather than split the team we agreed now was the time to stop. On the final day one of the surgeons berated us for paying so little attention to our Russian interpreter. She was an English teacher and not a doctor; while translating for the team she had witnessed terrible injury and tragedy, but never flinched or faltered. He was determined to strike up a conversation. Wishing to ask about her own experience of the earthquake, he asked: 'And did you feel the earth move?' To which she replied, 'even in Russia ... sometimes.' He blushed, she winked – we all smiled. So much tension eased, if only for a moment.

On our way back through Yerevan, we were approached by a British TV crew asking us to pose in the bar of a hotel, looking unused and frustrated. The story being run back home, they explained to us, was that the Russians were wasting all the foreign aid that was pouring in. I declined and moved the team on. If there was a lack of co-ordination it was more on the international side, and within a few years this experience led to the formation of the United Nations Disaster and Assessment Coordination Team (UNDAC), of which I was a founder member.

I left Armenia with a very heavy heart. And it wasn't just because of the terrible misery I had witnessed. On the contrary. The strength of human spirit shown by the survivors was inspiring. But that only served to amplify the frustration I felt at our failure in the face of so much need. Was the doing enough, in and of itself? We hadn't saved many lives, but we had extended the hand of friendship in times of trouble. We had given of ourselves. The flood of western aid workers through the iron curtain had mesmerised the Soviet authorities. 'We were taught you'd only ever come here to kill us,' people said to me many times, overawed by the magnitude and generosity shown to them by their enemies.

But was it nothing more than a grand gesture? And if so is that all bad? Can and should the softer, less tangible, social and political effects be factored into the final cost–benefit analysis? To counter the screaming self-doubt and self-criticism I became determined to do it better if I ever had the chance. So did the Swedes, the Austrians, the Italians and even the French, who in fairness had done it rather well. They were in first with a multidisciplinary team flown in by military aircraft. It could be done. The founder members of UNDAC contained many veterans of the Armenian earthquake, all determined to exorcise the ghosts of their failures by all doing it better next time.

Some years later when I was discussing with civil servants why the British Government seemed so slow to pick up on the lessons of Armenia, I was told I had made three very grave mistakes. The first was that on my return I had failed to say in interviews and in my writings that the British response was the best. My second mistake was worse: I had said the French were better. But my third mistake was the most serious of all. He said they knew I was right.

*

Late December 1988. Home. When I arrived back, life should have slowly got back to normal. But it didn't. On my first night at home, even before I'd unpacked, the phone rang. It was one of the team saying that the TV news was reporting that a jumbo jet had crashed over land and he was concerned we may be called upon to respond. I very much doubted this, as the UK had no national response for major incidents. Still, he made the point that the publicity surrounding our work in Armenia might just prompt a call on our services and I agreed he should at least alert the other members of the team. Meanwhile I rang RAF Valley in Anglesey. They had regularly helped SMART transport severely burned patients from distant hospitals into the regional burns unit in the hospital where I worked. I figured I was sufficiently well known to them to perhaps get more information. I was told they knew little more at this stage but if the team was required, they would be in touch. No sooner had I put the phone down than it rang again. 'This is RAF Edinburgh. A plane has crashed north of Carlisle. Two helicopters have been scrambled from RAF Valley for you and your team.' I was told to rendezvous at Manchester airport. By the time I'd confirmed it with the team there were blue lights flashing outside the window. My over-trousers and anorak still lying in the hall where I'd left them as my children smothered me with hugs on my return from Armenia. I picked them up ruefully and left the house in silence.

The helicopter journey to Lockerbie passed quickly and for the most part in silence. The crew had little more information to impart, other than that it was thought the plane might have crashed onto a petrol station in the town. As the helicopter began its descent I could see why. There was a huge bomb crater in the ground, still smoking, with intermittent bursts of flame lighting up the still night air. The surrounding roads were picked out from the blackness by winking blue lights, moving like fireflies from all directions to gather and stop in one central point. The helicopter had not fully settled itself on the ground when a policeman shouted to its opening doors for assistance. He took me to the edge of the crater into which he pointed at the smoking twisted embers of tree-like remains, left black and naked by the rush of fire. He and I both knew it wasn't a tree. It was to be the first of too many bodies that I would see that night.

I asked an officer in a patrol car to take us to the command and control centre. He couldn't. He was from Glasgow and had only just arrived at the scene. Moreover, the command and control centre had been changed, more than once, as the scale of the disaster unfolded. I introduced myself to the senior police officer, who in turn introduced me to the doctor in charge. He wasn't even a local doctor but was on holiday in the area. He had seen the plane crash, mounted the green light he carried in his car, and raced to the scene. He was newly qualified, in spite of his apparent age and bearing, and acknowledging his lack of training in emergency medicine, we agreed I should take over until the appearance of a more appropriate candidate – preferably local. It was late the following day before I could make the hand over.

We combed the fields in a bright moonlight that shone upon bodies and aircraft wherever they'd fallen. The pilot could be seen still strapped in his seat staring out onto an upturned world; his co-pilot savagely and incongruously replaced by the cold Scottish hillside. Rescue workers were pouring in and looking for medical support. No one was optimistic enough to imagine you survived a fall of 38,000 feet. But they were realistic enough to worry about debris, and even bodies, causing injury to those on the ground, and that identifying human remains might be very difficult. We did our best to spread ourselves amongst them. Our work was tireless. As well as searching the countryside for the fallen, we established a medical control centre alongside the command and control desks of the police, ambulance, and fire service. Additional information was sparse. We were expecting to see the response grow but it appeared muted.

Running parallel to this increasing activity on our part was a curious inertia at a higher level. We were in the early stages of a major incident response but where was everyone? True, the army was searching the hills for bodies, and helicopters were buzzing overhead. The firefighters and police were working flat out. But Malcolm Rifkind, the Scottish Secretary, had already been and gone by the time we got there – and we got there pretty quickly. Medical teams from Glasgow and Edinburgh hospitals had been mobilised then sent back home. The impression was of containment, postponement. Go home, get a good night's sleep and let's sort it all out in the morning. The response was scaled down to tick over until the morning light would allow the real work to begin. But this troubled us greatly. What to do when the local doctors have been quickly stood down, but you are asked to stay and given work to do? 'They're all dead, there's nothing more to do,' was the voice of officialdom. How were they so sure what had happened? If a bus had crashed off a bridge in Manchester and clearly no one could have survived it, we wouldn't have sent people away advising them we would sort it all out in the morning. But when a plane crashed in Scotland this is what they did. Lockerbie was an awful experience made worse a thousand times by the feeling that we were intruding on something we weren't supposed to see. In retrospect, they must have known before we got there that it was bomb.

As the night went on the command and control centre took shape. We were asked to accompany teams searching the fields for bodies, but were instructed to leave them where they were. This would be a criminal investigation from the outset.

The feeling of abandonment was demonstrated graphically when deep in the night I went to discuss a problem with a an official. As a result of the 'wait until dawn' policy, he was now left alone in a school room, sat at a school desk, with a single phone in its centre. There was some confusion over the body-labelling system which I wanted to bring to the attention of the authorities. Some had no labels; others had several. He was obviously stressed, tired and uncertain. 'Look, it's simple. We have prenumbered labels matching the number of passengers,' he said pointing to a box. 'They are tagged to a body and that way we will know when the box is empty, they have all been located.' As he realised the labels were here on his desk and not there in the fields, he simply slumped forward and hit his head on the phone; he could take no more, it was all too much. 'Don't worry,' I said, putting my arm around his shoulders, we can easily start again.

Word went around that a contingent of bereaved relatives from America were flying in overnight, heralding a bitter expansion of this already awful human tragedy. Their impending arrival spurred us on. We were sustained throughout the night by hot food cooked by a band of good-hearted volunteers. Prince Andrew arrived, and in different times was very well received by all, but especially the soldiers. I was eating a sausage sandwich when he walked past me, refusing to shake my grubby hands. The arrival of Margaret Thatcher did not go down so well. When news of her coming went around, the mood was angry and openly hostile. Rescue teams and soldiers alike made it clear that they thoroughly disapproved of politicians cashing in on human tragedy. The Royal Family could visit; that's what they did, and it was both expected and appreciated. Margaret Thatcher, on the other hand, was a politician and not particularly popular at that time as I recall. It was clear that if she came into the centre where we were gathered her reception would at the very least be somewhat muted, and there was a good risk it would be openly and vocally hostile. All in all, it would not achieve the good media coverage for which she'd come. So instead she stayed well away from the workers, far out of range, and we all breathed a little easier.

Before the arrival of the dignitaries, dawn had broken on a town besieged. News reporters were scurrying everywhere looking for the saddest, most grotesque image their editors would dare to print. A passenger still strapped in their seat but now on a roof, was a particular focus of attention. Earlier that morning my team and I had stood in a hall and listened to a senior police officer, looking clean and fresh from sleep, tug at his crisp brown leather gloves and tell us, without irony, that the real work was about to begin. The eyes of the world would be upon us he said, and he was confident we would rise to the task. The officer again reminded us that this was a criminal investigation. All bodies were to be left where they fell. Tagged and numbered, but not to be moved. In time they would be photographed and videoed before transport to the mortuary. These words were in my head as the growing light shone down on the bodies embedded in the roof, on the hill, over the town. I imagined residents of the town looking up at this modern Calvary and how it would become a beacon for the world's press. So, we took her down. I walked back along the street and a radio journalist asked, 'What's the worst thing you've seen?', as a microphone was thrust, unasked for, into my face. 'You,' I said. It was never broadcast.

The residents of Lockerbie suffered terribly. A plane fell out of the sky, killing their neighbours and changing their town forever. Into the midst of such sudden and terrible torment human beings will always try to force normality. To will the horror away and make life as it was seconds before disaster. I saw a man pushing his way through crowds of media and rescuers to bang on the door of the local shop. Why wasn't it open? He needed his milk and morning paper. He already knew the news, but he was screaming for normality.

It wasn't just me who failed to leave the dead where they lay. People found bodies in the street, some small enough for them to be thrust in my arms. Others stood frozen, staring out of their bedroom windows at a white flash that had flown past their window, bounced off their garden and now nesting in a tree. Bodies were everywhere. Clothes torn off by the rush of the speeding air, limbs concertinaed into their torsos by the huge impact of the fall. Whoever planted that bomb committed multiple, terrible murders. They blasted people, young and old alike, out of the sky and into the freezing air. Bodies hung like washing, draped forwards and backwards over fences and trees.

Most poignant were the Christmas presents. The spirits of the victims lay trapped in the brightly coloured and still unopened parcels scattered across the hillside, in gardens, and crushed beneath our feet as we climbed over them to reach the passengers. They screamed of the misery unfolding in hundreds of homes: of joyful anticipation turned suddenly and viciously to despair. The horror of the act lay not in the bodies themselves but more in the everlasting heartache they heralded. The horror lay in the heart of a man who could blot out his own experience of love and loss and inflict so much pain upon his fellow human beings. The horror lay in the man who remembered his own joy and suffering and still placed the bomb.

We laboured on throughout a heavy and painful day. The need for medical support to those continuing to search for remains was gradually taken up by staff from a local hospital. They had been prepared to receive casualties but had been stood down almost as soon as the incident unfolded, having been told they were all dead. I contacted psychologists to assist rescue workers and townsfolk alike, and they responded quickly and efficiently. One of my closest colleagues, a consultant of many years standing, was severely distressed by what he saw. 'But why this?' I asked him, 'when you have already seen so much.' He spoke for all of us when he said, 'It was not just seeing so many dead people, though that was bad enough, but seeing them against the day to day background of an ordinary town and not in the artificial environment of a ward. It was just too real.'

As the day drew to a close and our duties were either complete or by now taken over by locals, we made ready to go home. I went to search out the RAF team who'd brought us there to find out from them when we might be taken back. The crew who had brought us had now gone. The crews who had now replaced them informed me with frank, emotionless military logic that they were posted to Lockerbie, where they would remain until ordered otherwise. They could offer no help or advice about the return journey. The words 'we are not a taxi service' ended the conversation. For the first time I felt the overwhelming tiredness of a day and a night without sleep. I couldn't argue. If I were to articulate the injustice of it all I would either boil in rage or more likely melt into tears. I gathered what strength I had left and did what all British do in a crisis. I asked a policeman. I poured out my plight and he didn't flinch. He looked down at me, standing there in my fireproof overalls and with no sense of irony, and definitely no humour, suggested I might get the bus. 'But I have no money' I said, turning out my pockets to show nothing but a rolled-up rouble. Now irritated that he was being drawn into a problem he couldn't or just didn't want to solve he snapped 'Where do you live?'. 'Manchester' I replied. With a show of obvious relief, he declared me 'homeless and penniless in Scotland' and 'that's social services,' he beamed triumphantly.

I gathered the team, and we joined a queue of townsfolk seeking emergency assistance from the state. When I reached the front of the queue, I retold the tale of our predicament and once again received no word of solace. It was duly noted that we were all officially homeless and penniless in Scotland. 'But you do have somewhere to stay if we get you there tonight?'. 'Just turning up has always worked before,' I said. And with that he looked up the cost of a second-class single railway ticket from Carlisle to Manchester and counted the exact cost in pounds and pennies into each of our open hands. When I asked how we might get to Carlisle l was told again to get the bus. At this point a quiet elderly man stepped forwards and said, 'I'll get the school bus and it will be my pleasure to drive you to Carlisle.'

At the start of that month we had been sat on a coach, climbing a hill to catastrophe in a foreign land. At the top of the hill we had comforted ourselves with the thought that such terrible troubles only ever happened elsewhere, that our homeland would always be spared. At the end of the month we were back on a coach coming down from the hills, where the unthinkable had happened, and this time on home turf.

We sat in uncharacteristic silence on the coach to Carlisle. Our shabby treatment at the hands of the authorities had failed to raise one word of protest in a group not normally known for its reticence. Such was our weariness and sorrow. The stationmaster at Carlisle station took pity on our dishevelled state and the attention our clothing and equipment was attracting and let us wait in a private room. Ignoring what it said on our tickets, the guard on the train gave us a first-class compartment all to ourselves.

In less than a month my life had been transformed. It was my wedding anniversary the day I was in Lockerbie. It was Christmas eve on my return home. The combination of Armenia and Lockerbie completely and utterly flattened me. At night in bed I woke terrified and sweating, suffocating in a pile of dead bodies. I lay silent on the sofa all over Christmas, ignoring my young family as they tried to enjoy the festivities; unable to move or think through a thick fog of imagery and an unbearable weight of sadness. I realised I had to make a choice. Resolve never to do anything like this again, bury it, put it all behind me, and spare myself and my family; or make it my life's work and do it properly. For better or worse, I chose the latter.

4.

Besieged

Sarajevo

The Siege of Sarajevo began on 5 April 1992 and ran until 29 February 1996. Not long after the Siege began, I offered our medical team SMART to the Overseas Development Administration (ODA), at the time the overseas aid arm of the Foreign and Commonwealth Office of the UK Government, to support any British aid effort to the beleaguered city. The ODA would initially reject the offer, but finally on 14 July 1992 I was asked to carry out an assessment mission in Sarajevo on their behalf, leaving that same day. So sudden was the move that the first my brother Michael heard of it was on the car radio when Prime Minister John Major announced our deployment to the House of Commons.

Unsure of what we might find, I assembled a team with both experience of previous disasters and also the skills and experience to facilitate an assessment of needs in the hospitals of Sarajevo. We also had the personnel and equipment for lifesaving surgery and other treatments should they be required. The team was fully equipped and ready to leave by 5pm that day. While passing through Manchester airport an enterprising ODA civil servant had persuaded a somewhat surprised, but quickly willing, Serbo-

Croat speaking immigration officer to accompany us on our quest.

We arrived in Zagreb in the small hours of the morning. British troops working with the UN unloaded the plane and we were taken in a UN vehicle to a hotel where we were greeted by newspaper reporters. They were pushing hard for detailed information and interviews. I told them we were there to assess the situation, but I noted at the time that they 'clearly appeared hostile to the mission'. Why there was such a reaction to a group of volunteer NHS health workers was unclear to me at the time, but it has been an intermittent feature of my work in later, similar missions. It appears to me that by working closely with a government department, even as an unpaid volunteer carrying out humanitarian work and risking your life in a dangerous environment, some of the press have difficulty in dissociating this from the activities of politicians and civil servants. You become 'fair game'.

If it isn't already hard enough to be setting out into an active war zone and placing yourself unarmed between the warring factions, then the actions of some of the press can at times do nothing to ease these difficulties. But you must also sometimes contend with the internal machinations of your own government. A few hours after our arrival I was greeted in the lobby of the hotel by someone who said they were a representative of the Foreign and Commonwealth Office (FCO) and couldn't see why we were there. Sporting a fashionable safari suit, they said the FCO had been informed by the ICRC that they had been into Sarajevo and assessed there to be 'world class' hospitals and staff, but a shortage of supplies. However, they thought they might be able to find 'something for the team to do' in Zagreb. These words echoed those of the British ambassador at the airport in Moscow on our way to

Armenia a few years before, offering to find us 'something to do' in Moscow instead. That time the offer was also accompanied by their reassurance that 'they would never need to know back home'. Tensions between the ODA, later the Department for International Development (DFID) and the FCO remained as long as I worked on overseas humanitarian deployments. Politics, diplomacy and humanitarian aid are uneasy bedfellows.

Not knowing if these new orders superseded our earlier instructions, I rang my contact at ODA, who advised me to ignore the FCO representative and prepare to proceed to Sarajevo that day. I was buggered if I would turn back now, so I agreed. The last UN aid flight into Sarajevo that day was at 1pm and was fortuitously operated by the RAF. They would fly us into the city. I travelled with an experienced plastic and reconstructive surgeon, Dr Stewart Watson, who could provide further specialist assessment, and our interpreter, arriving at the airport with fifteen minutes to spare only to find that a bureaucratic cock-up or some other connivance had denied us the paperwork to board the taxiing plane. I suspected foul play and the machinations of our friend in the safari suit. My suspicions were strengthened when immediately after the plane had taken off without us aboard, our British contact at the airport produced from his top pocket the missing authorisation to fly. However, all was not lost. I'd heard an Italian Air Force plane might be making a brief stop on a round trip from Ancona in Italy via Sarajevo, so decided to wait. An Italian paediatrician who was working for UNICEF had arrived for the Italian plane and he approached me. He said he'd witnessed the shenanigans and in solidarity, doctor to doctor, offered to try and get us on their plane.

The pilot kept its engines running as our new ally made his way across the tarmac. He'd asked us to stand by the hangar doors while he ran to speak with the captain. He waved from the plane door indicating for us to join him, and we ran as fast as we could before anyone could stop us. The Italian crew was prepared to take us without any official papers and were most welcoming, dubbing us the 'invisible men.' I noted that as we approached Sarajevo Airport, they did not employ the steep landing dive to avoid missile attack I had been told to expect, and experienced on the later airlifts. They instead chose what seemed to me to be a normal shallow approach. Six weeks later the plane was shot down and my newfound Italian friends were killed. The wreckage of the plane was eventually made into a monument at Ancona Airport, from where I flew in and out of Sarajevo for much of the remaining years of the war. I always stopped to pay my respects and remember their bravery, warmth, and kindness.

We arrived in Sarajevo in early evening to a soundtrack of gunfire and shelling. Being a civilian team, we had been unable to equip ourselves with flak jackets and were not offered them on arrival. However, we found some ourselves in the UNHCR hanger and asked to borrow them. We were given transport into the city in a UNHCR 'soft skinned' (unarmoured) 4x4 with an armoured personal carrier (APC) as escort. We were taken to UNPROFOR, United Nations Protection Force, housed in the Post Office and Telecommunications (PTT) building in Sarajevo. I located and introduced myself to the remarkable Major Vanessa Lloyd Davies, the British medical officer for UNPROFOR, and spent that first evening with her discussing the situation. Like all of us, she was deeply affected by her experiences in Sarajevo. As a young army medical officer with, until then, little exposure to the clinical management of major injury, the day before we met she had been required to care for five children who had been horribly injured by mortar fire outside the UN building. She had huge responsibilities. Soldiers were frequently hit by snipers – even in the car park of the UN headquarters – and it was she, a young, newly qualified, non-specialist doctor, who was responsible for their immediate care. Vanessa Lloyd-Davies took her own life some years later, for reasons unknown. Her experiences in Sarajevo, and the horribly injured children she cared for, featured in her obituary.

Once in the PTT we were offered a bed for the night in an empty room on the fourth floor. The room appeared to us to be rather exposed to sniper fire and shelling, but we were able to arrange some sturdy tables to shield us from any falling glass as we slept on the floor in our sleeping bags. The building was in a terrible state. It had been damaged by shellfire and its water supply was poor. The toilets were broken and blocked, overflowing with faecal waste. Gun and shellfire rattled and thudded through the night, some of it alarmingly close. As shells from both Serbs and Croats crisscrossed overhead, a British soldier reassured us that they were not directed at our building and we could ease ourselves off to sleep by trying to work out from where the shells were coming and where they might be heading. It didn't work. Later I was able to witness the arrival of the French Foreign Legion when they took over the command of the PTT from the force that was there initially. It was transformational. These disciplined, scary guys made them clean up the place before leaving, including the toilets, and importantly implemented proper security. The meals also improved dramatically, and included wine with the evening meal.

The next day, Major Lloyd Davies organised our journey to Sarajevo's 'Kosevo' hospital by armoured personal carrier. En route we were surprised to stop at the now infamous Holiday Inn, situated on 'Sniper Alley', where young French aid workers had been shot and killed only the day before. They had been sat outside in the sun, singing and playing guitar. This dangerous detour we learned was to pick up a 'Harley Street' doctor who had driven alone from the coastal town of Split to Sarajevo on behalf of a private charity and the *Sunday Times*, he said. I don't know what he did at the hospital, and I never heard of him again. I couldn't decide whether he had been incredibly brave, extremely foolhardy, or simply naïve. I'm sure people have thought the same about me.

On arrival at the hospital we met its medical director who gave us a prepared list of their needs. I received similar lists when carrying out assessment missions in Serbia and Montenegro on behalf of WHO. There were, he said, long-term funding problems for their health service, as well as the acute problems caused by the war. He was requesting very high tech equipment, including dialysis machines, though they lacked the means to conduct the most basic biochemical tests essential to monitor dialysis. He wanted many very expensive and non-essential drugs, and appeared quite out of touch with the true needs of the hospital. Over the years I became familiar with these wish lists from the 'big man' (they were always men) in charge of the hospital. I suspected they were collecting expensive equipment for their private clinics. In the early days of the war they might have thought it wouldn't last long so were stockpiling for after the aid circus had moved on.

Having our own interpreter was extremely valuable. I've always found a local interpreter wherever I've travelled, but their loyalties can be mixed and when dealing with oppressive governments and gangsters (sometimes one and the same thing), what they translate will be what they think is safest for them to say. But we were on safe ground with our co-opted immigration officer. A tour of the wards revealed the most urgent needs to be basic items: dressings, urine catheters, Plaster of Paris and basic medicines. The operating theatres in the Institute of Traumatology needed more sophisticated support, including anaesthetic drugs, a reliable anaesthetic machine and a working diathermy to cauterise blood vessels during surgery. The Institute was heavily guarded by Bosnian militia who were very suspicious of our presence. Our interpreter intervened when my bushy and (then) very black beard led them to noisily ask why the Chetnik (Serbian militia from the Second World War) was here? We moved off sharpish.

On arrival at the airport in Sarajevo we'd been greeted by Larry Hollingsworth of UNHCR, who went on to become the face of Sarajevo for the media over the coming months and a good friend to me. He'd told us that they had originally taken aid directly to the hospitals but no-one there would unload it. Instead they were told to take it to one of four stockpiles from where it would be distributed. The true fate of this early aid to the hospitals appeared to be unknown. Whether it too was being hoarded in case the aid dried up (a not uncommon phenomenon), or being diverted elsewhere, perhaps to the frontline, was unknown. My later experience of working in the hospital suggested the latter my be true, but I didn't reveal my suspicions. If I had the aid funding we had might cease, and nobody would get help. This was but one of many compromises I was to make over the years.

Other compromises, omissions and white lies were necessary. On my return to the PTT I had to pretend to be a member of staff to use the UNICEF office satellite phone to brief the ODA and fax through pages of medical supplies for purchase in the UK. My lack of a UN ID badge raised suspicions, but the Foreign Legion were weeks away from arriving and security was still loose. I confidently signed for the use of the phone and left. In fact, it was some months before I secured a UN ID badge. I once got through a Serb check-point with a group of UN workers by flashing a Diner's Club card – blue, like the UN ID. The first night I tried to get into the UN building after the arrival of the Legionnaires I was not so lucky. There was a queue in the yard outside while they were now metic-ulously checking everyone's ID. We were outside, exposed to snipers and keen to get inside to relative safety. I still had no UN ID but worse still, this time I didn't have my passport, having forgotten it at Ancona airport on the flight out. A whispered chat with a colleague further up the queue who looked about the same age and was bearded like me, and he agreed to pass his passport down the queue after he'd been checked in. I frantically memorised his date and place of birth and managed to get safely inside. I foiled another checkpoint by walking in the middle of a group of UN workers, looking straight ahead, before embarking a plane. My colleagues brought my passport to me in Ancona and I could get back into Italy. I've never forgotten a passport again.

*

Uncoordinated action under pressure always leads to waste. At the airport on our way out after this first assessment mission we iden-tified four mechanical ventilators in a consignment of aid from Kuwait that had been there for several days. Kosevo hospital had a desperate need for ventilators but the non-medical staff at the airport were unaware of their significance and had consigned them to the stockpile. As a parting action before we flew back to Zagreb we were able to arrange for their direct transport to the hospital. In Armenia I saw medical equipment rotting on the airfield just as I did here in Sarajevo. We would see it again and again over the coming years. Aid sent to disasters without first securing its passage to the intended recipients is destined to disappear somewhere on its journey.

Our flight out was this time courtesy of the RAF and we boarded with no subterfuge or resistance. We were met in Zagreb by Dr Mukesh Kapila, who later found fame for his courageous work in Darfur, but was then working for the ODA. He helped us transmit our full list of requirements for the hospitals through to London that night. I still work with Mukesh today.

There too I met with Sir Donald Acheson, then the former Chief Medical Officer in the UK and now Special Representative of the Regional Director of the World Health Organisation. The Serbs had complained to the UN that I was only assessing needs on the Bosnian side, he explained. So, he handed me my next mission, to undertake a similar assessment in Serbia and Montenegro for WHO, including Kosovo, where I was to spend a year some seven years later. I was home for only a week before I was granted special leave by the hospital where I was a full time NHS A&E Consultant, and left for Serbia and Montenegro.

5.

Maybe Airlines

Kosovo / Serbia and Montenegro

The situation in Serbia was highly unstable. International sanctions meant that there were no flights into Belgrade, so I would have to go by train from Budapest and through dangerous territory near the border. I had read an article in a Sunday paper just before leaving that described how militia held up and robbed the trains from Budapest as they entered Vojvodina in northern Serbia. I took an early morning flight from Manchester to Geneva before a connecting flight to Budapest that evening. My seat neighbour was on a business trip and asked me the purpose of my visit to Geneva. She fell silent when I told her. She looked at me with genuine sorrow and wished me luck, but I could see she thought luck would not be enough for me to make it out alive.

Despite the nature of my mission I was genuinely awestruck to find myself for the first time walking into the Geneva headquarters of the World Health Organisation, and proud to be taking up a consultant post. However, such positive feelings quickly ebbed away when I was told nobody was available to meet with me: they were busy in meetings, discussing the crisis in Yugoslavia. The irony was not lost on me. So, I waited all morning and then on into the afternoon. I busied myself by signing my contract and getting my blue UN passport (laissez-passer). Come late afternoon I was told the security briefing I had been promised would not now go ahead. Instead I was handed an envelope stuffed full of banknotes and told that when I arrived in Budapest I was to get on the early morning Orient Express from Budapest to Belgrade. I was to get to the station several hours beforehand so that I could purchase every seat in a carriage and lock the doors at both ends. This, they said, was to protect me from the raids on the train that I already knew were a hazard of the journey.

In Budapest my attempts to buy every seat in a carriage were met with a combination of incredulity and faint amusement. In any event the train was already almost full. So, I got my one ticket and boarded the train. Everyone in the busy carriage was friendly. There were bags and suitcases everywhere and even live chickens in cages on people's knees. I felt my anxieties ease, but not for long. As we were about to cross from Hungary into Serbia, the Serbian police boarded the train. They were very aggressive with barking German Shepherd dogs straining at the leash. They asked to see our documents and when I handed over my UN laissez-passer; the officer looked at it in utter distain and became very angry, remonstrating with his colleagues about UN sanctions and jabbing his finger at me. I thought I was about to be arrested. In a moment of inspiration, or panic, I fumbled for, and flourished, my British passport. His frown turned to a slow smile as he took it from me. 'I would advise you to not use the blue passport in Serbia, my friend,' he said softly. 'Use your British passport. The British are our allies.' This was early in the conflict and the Serbs were yet to learn otherwise.

I arrived safely in Belgrade in the early evening. I was met at the station by a Serbian official and taken by car to a government building. My itinerary for the two weeks of my mission was explained. I would be travelling with a Serbian public health doctor and driver and would visit health facilities throughout Serbia Montenegro and Kosovo. They checked my passport (British) but I wouldn't let them keep it, holding it close to me at all times. Early the following morning we set off on our serpiginous journey. We visited at least two health facilities each day, sleeping in a different small hotel each night. I had no contact with the outside world.

When travelling through remote mountainous country I could almost forget about the war. Bizarrely we found ourselves once behind a touring caravan with Swiss number plates, oblivious to the war that had erupted into their vacation. I was to experience a similar incongruity towards the end of my time in Bosnia. I managed to get a flight out of Split in a now peaceful Croatia to find myself on a plane packed with returning holidaymakers who passed no comment at me loading my helmet and flak jacket into the overhead locker.

But the war was in fact never very far away. At one point we got so close to the front line that a nurse from a hospital we visited and who spoke English pulled me quietly to one side and told me that the route they were intending to take me was far too dangerous. People had been killed there only the day before, she whispered, with a frightened look on her face. But I had no choice; I was entirely in the hands of my Serbian minders. As it happened, we did not come under attack, although we could hear gunfire nearby. This pattern of imminent threat, anxiety, and then anti-climax was repeated endlessly throughout the coming years. I learned that the constant threat of danger, if sustained over a prolonged period, is in many ways worse and more damaging than intermittent heightened episodes of obvious imminent threat. It certainly was for me.

We also visited Kosovo. The parallel system that the ethnic Albanians had instituted in protest against the Serbs meant that government hospitals were now staffed mainly by disgruntled Serbians from Belgrade who had been forcibly transferred to work in the region. Meanwhile the Albanians ran makeshift hospitals, including surgical operating theatres, in their homes, while the government hospitals treated ethnic Serbs and those Albanians who couldn't be managed in the makeshift parallel system. When I worked in Kosovo some years later, after the NATO intervention, Albanian doctors told me with pride how they would try to expand their clinical knowledge by getting tip-offs about 'interesting cases' in the Clinical Centre and pretending to be visitors to examine them. As romantic as this sounded I knew from observation of their limited clinical skills that the training they got in the parallel system was woefully inadequate and the medical degrees they awarded themselves did not stack up alongside those from other European medical schools. This caused me problems when the international community, including WHO, was keen to recognise the Albanian medical staff and their home-made qualifications in order to get the health service quickly back on its feet. As head of the hospital in Pristina I had to caution against a wholesale accept-ance on the grounds of patient safety.

Kosovo was clearly already on its knees. The hospitals were in disrepair and in need of equipment and medicines. Livestock roamed the grounds outside, brushing their way past the surgical linen drying on lines. In a hotel lobby in Pristina I again felt the threat of murmurings aimed against me. Heavyset young men, Albanian in origin, clearly associated me with my Serb minder who moved me away and advised me to go to my room. I locked the door and did not come out until breakfast.

I made daily notes on a small electronic personal organiser, completing my final report for submission to WHO by the time I was back in Belgrade. After the two weeks of the mission was up, I was driven back to government buildings in Belgrade where a minister demanded I hand over the device. 'We know you've been writing your report.' he said, 'and we want to see what you will be recommending to WHO before you leave Belgrade.' I told him my report was for WHO only. They could share it with them later if they wished, I explained, but my duty was to give my views directly to WHO. He was very angry and demanded that I hand it over immediately. I refused. The Serbs wanted outside aid, but at that stage of the conflict, what I saw and heard was evidence of a chronically neglected health service rather than an acute lack of drugs and equipment brought on by these few months of war. My Serb aggressor, I was sure, would know this from the reports of my discussions and questioning from my minder and was I guess desperate to ensure that any report that went in reflected what they wanted more than what they needed. But unless I opened the device he couldn't get the information himself, even if he took it forcibly, and this clearly frustrated him. I was very anxious but stood my ground. My anxiety progressed to fear as the day dragged on. I was left alone in the room: no food, no water, no toilet. Periodically different people would come in and demand that I hand over the report. Their manner became increasingly threatening, and although ultimately I was not physically harmed, I felt in grave danger and completely alone. As evening approached, I assumed that the verbal threats would likely become more tangible, and that I would certainly be incarcerated overnight. I was confronted yet again. 'Are you really not going to share the report?' he shouted into my face. 'No,' I said. Having held out for so long it was probably more stubbornness than anything now that made me continue to refuse. I'd already worked out that WHO would inevitably share the report and so I could save myself the bother and possible pain. But I didn't. I knew too that another assessment team was on its way. Towards the end of the two weeks I'd learned from my minder that WHO would soon be sending in a more comprehensive team and that my mission, dangerous as it was, was merely a holding measure. I felt terribly used – used to the point of tears – but determined to finish the mission as diligently as I could and hand over the report to Geneva, unadulterated, whether or not they still needed it.

'In that case you may as well go,' he conceded. Was this some sort of trap? I assumed that there had been calls to and from WHO all that day and he was now happy that he would get the report as soon as I got back to Geneva, or whatever the next team produced. I pushed my luck and asked if I could get a lift to the railway station. 'Dear me, no!' he said. 'Don't you know that train journey is far too dangerous? There are bandits who attack it! My driver will take you to the Hungarian border.' We drove through the night to a border crossing where my British passport saw me safely out of Serbia and into Hungary. I got an early morning flight into Geneva and handed in my report. Without so much as a debrief I arranged a flight home, to start back at work for the NHS the next day.

*

But before I left Geneva, I met again with Sir Donald Acheson, erstwhile Chief Medical Officer in the UK. He was a remarkable man and became a good friend, inviting me to his inauguration as President of the British Medical Association some years later. Now, in his retirement, he was the WHO special representative in Zagreb.

He was interested in the work that I had done in Sarajevo and in Serbia and I filled him in on what I had seen and learned. He asked me if I could arrange to stand in for him for a few weeks while he returned to the UK to brief the Prime Minister, amongst other things. Once again, all those I worked with were very supportive, and shortly afterwards I returned to Zagreb as acting Special Representative for WHO.

I relished the opportunity to travel throughout the conflict areas and gain more first-hand knowledge of the situation, but staff were insistent that I stay office-bound for the two weeks I was there. Sir Donald was newly appointed and always travelling which meant that a backlog of administrative tasks had built up. So, I shelved my ambitions and served my short time in Zagreb as a bureaucrat. The work was surprisingly interesting and showed me the depth of foundations required to support complex deployments. Medical staff from frontline facilities would make their way to Zagreb and ask WHO to supply them with drugs. I remember going with one such applicant to the WHO warehouse, where the manager told me we couldn't possibly give out emergency stocks to him as someone more needy may come along. If we kept giving them out, he said, we wouldn't have any left. I explained to him that the stocks were there precisely for this and it was our job to replenish them. This conflict between storing medical equipment and drugs for worse times ahead and using them to meet immediate needs is a recurring conflict in emergency and disaster management. The doctor had risked life and limb through battlefields to get to WHO for help. I gave him what he asked for and we successfully replenished the stocks.

I enjoyed my time in Zagreb. The war was no longer in the city unlike my first visit a few weeks earlier when air raids were still a feature. The staff I worked with were pleasant and helpful. I even had my own car and driver. Which raised another problem. While putting equipment into the boot I saw a detachable illuminated taxi sign. I took the driver for a coffee and asked him to explain and reminded him that he was paid by WHO to drive a WHO owned vehicle for WHO business. However, he said he had an extended family to support and his earnings were not great. He wanted to earn as much as he could in these troubled times and so was moon-lighting with the WHO vehicle as a taxi in the evenings. So, what to do? I could sack him and recruit another driver. But he was a good driver and reliable. What was the real harm? The WHO markings on the side of the vehicle were detachable and removed when acting as a taxi. What are you going to do he asked me? 'Nothing.' I said, 'as long as nobody else finds out.' They didn't.

*

Again, I went back to my work in the trauma centre at the North Staffordshire hospital. This constant moving between peace and war was extremely stressful. When in Sarajevo I worried about my family but also about my job. There were times when I was contacted by satellite phone to remind me that I was needed for the on-call rota. The airlift in and out of Sarajevo was very unreliable and known affectionately as 'maybe' airlines. Maybe you would get a seat on the plane. Maybe the weather would allow it to take off. Maybe the Serbs wouldn't shoot it down. Maybe the weather at your destination would allow it to land. I couldn't ever guarantee if or when I could be back in the UK. My colleagues were very accommodating, but it was a source of constant tension. Until matters became more regulated, the UN troops would stamp your passport with 'Maybe Airlines' – a souvenir I still treasure.

6.

Operation Phoenix

Macedonia / Sarajevo

As the winter set in I was asked by WHO to set up their office in Sarajevo. I took further leave from the NHS and headed again for Geneva and then into Bosnia. But how to get in? The airlift was not functioning because of threats to shoot it down, so I had to try and get in overland. I flew into Split in Croatia but found no help there. Not so much hostility as indifference from the local WHO office. Determined to complete the mission, I did learn where the ODA land convoy would be leaving from, and somehow persuaded a visitor to the office to give me a lift. Sadly, by the time we got there it had left. By now my new friend was as determined as me to not be defeated and we raced along the main road out of town assuming that would be their route, and it was. We caught them up. He pulled his car in front of the lead truck to make it stop and I got out. Fortunately, there were no armed guards on the convoy, otherwise the outcome may have been very different. I climbed up to the driver's side of the cab and introduced myself as a fellow Brit working for WHO. Would they please give me a lift into Sarajevo? Without much reflection the head of the convoy, who until recently had been working in a bank in the UK, agreed. He held out his hand and I climbed into the cab and sat next to him. I had my way in. There was a Wild West atmosphere in those early days among those volunteering on this the frontline.

We progressed up the mountain until darkness fell. The Serbs held us at their checkpoint and went through all its contents. I slept on the floor of a deserted café, freezing in the depths of a Sarajevo winter. At first light the truck drivers lit fires under the frozen diesel tanks to get the fuel to a consistency where it would flow through the engine and take us through the menace of the Serb military and into the besieged and sorry city. The convoy ended its journey at the bakery in the centre of town and once again I had to fend for myself. It was extremely dangerous for me to be standing out there in the open where snipers would pick you off like ducks at a funfair. I managed to stop a passing UN vehicle and persuade the driver to give me a lift to the UN headquarters at the PTT building where I set about establishing a WHO office. I had great support from local doctors including Dr Jganjac, who found international fame when advocating for the medical evacuation of his young patient, Irma. He would meet me outside the perimeter of the UN building, barred from entry as a local, and we would travel in his beat-up old VW to the hospital. One morning when we couldn't get through the safer back route, we hurtled down Sniper Alley singing 'Que Sera Sera' at the top of our voices, in a state of fear and exhilaration at the risk we were taking.

When the office was running, and more staff were en route, I headed home again, leaving behind the profound greyness, emptiness, sparseness and sorrow that was Sarajevo. Its frightened, wounded people, starving in their battered homes and hideouts, without water and electricity, were etched deeply into my brain, and clashed violently with the blinding brightness of Zagreb. The city had recovered quickly from its war and now with Christmas lights and decorations. Well fed, happy people, strolled around, not running from snipers, peering into shops bursting with food and gifts. The sheer normality of it all overwhelmed me. Inside I was screaming at every person I saw, asking how they could ignore what was happening so close to them: to those who were only recently their fellow countrymen. I managed to garner enough calm to buy a bottle of wine and retreated to my hotel room. I felt better in its relative simplicity. It felt less of a betrayal of those I'd left behind in that godforsaken city. I ate an army ration pack I'd saved from the PTT building and I drank the wine. In an act of self-pity and sheer desolation I sang the words of 'Away in a Manger' to myself and cried. And cried. I slept on the floor, as I had in Sarajevo. Early next morning I flew home.

*

Was my work in Sarajevo humanitarian in all its guises? I don't know, but I'm confident it was the right thing to do.

In a situation with asymmetric needs, it is always a struggle to maintain your impartiality. Today, there are four principles that define humanitarian actions – humanity, neutrality, impartiality, and independence. And of these four, it is the first, the imperative that human suffering must be addressed wherever it is found, that drives much of humanitarian intervention. I'm confident I maintained my impartiality in Sarajevo, as elsewhere. But neutrality in the face of suffering and overwhelming injustice? I'm not sure. By the end of my time in Sarajevo I prioritised the Bosnian community over the Serbs, having witnessed for myself the huge disparity in need between the two communities, and that the cause of so much continuing suffering in one community was the actions of the other. Social justice would surely demand that the greatest benefit be to the least advantaged.

I've acted independently whenever I can, partly by setting up my own organisation, though the ability to do so is increasingly threatened in the face of complex emergencies. But how far one is truly independent when funded by others, particularly governments, is always open to question. In Sarajevo the programme I ran was funded solely by the British government – part of a wider British aid programme that was the outcome of an even wider political process towards bolstering a ceasefire; brokering a peace; and preventing the war from spilling over into neighbouring countries. Did I, could I, maintain my independence all along that line? And, if I didn't, was it wrong?

In March 1993, I was asked by the ODA to travel to what was by then the Former Republic of Yugoslavia Macedonia. Its infrastructure was poor, tragically reflected in the loss of a Palair Macedonian airlines aircraft that crashed shortly after take-off from Skopje Airport, killing 83 of the 97 persons on board, a week or so before I was due to leave. The crash and its aftermath hung heavily over the city, and especially the medical staff I spoke with, many of whom had dealt with its human consequences.

Macedonia had not long since declared its independence, and so far had avoided being drawn into the wars now burning across its neighbours. The rest of Europe and NATO were determined to keep it that way, and supporting the incumbent government was viewed as one way of maintaining stability and containing in its borders the ethnic tensions then tearing the rest of the Balkans apart. Dissatisfaction with the delivery of healthcare by any government is always a key component of any wider dissatisfaction and preventing it from failing completely was seen as a priority by the West. This was the basis of my mission.

Although Macedonia had largely avoided the bloody fallout from the breakup of the Yugoslav Republic, this small new country of fewer than 2 million people, could not avoid its economic consequences. These were reflected across the health system, and particularly in the paucity of essential drugs, both in the hospitals and in the community. I made detailed recommendations and a substantial medical aid package was delivered to the Macedonian government shortly afterwards. I am confident that many people in genuine need were helped by this intervention, but was it humanitarian? Was it neutral and impartial and was I acting independently? And was it fair? If looking through the lens of social justice solely at Macedonia, then I am confident it would see the greatest benefit going to the least advantaged with what was an equitable supply of drugs. But widening the field of vision to the former Yugoslavia as a whole, the people of Macedonia were not the most disadvantaged, and if looking across the world, they were comparatively advantaged. If you can't help everyone, should you help no one, or simply help those you can? This was my opportunity to include healthcare in the wider economic package put together to help stabilise the country: a package that may even have worked. Certainly, Macedonia didn't fall into chaos; and the war didn't spill over into a NATO country, thus avoiding the catastrophic bonfire that might have been ignited. My work in Macedonia, though, proved to be but a trial run for my involvement in what was to become a much larger use of aid as a political stabiliser, and a bigger test of my independence.

In December 1992, while I was working in the emergency department of the trauma hospital in Sarajevo, the intensive care unit on the floor above me was holed by an anti-aircraft shell. It went through the wall on one side of the ward, between the beds, and out through the wall on the other side, but remarkably did not explode. Not long afterwards, early one morning I was woken from snatched sleep, by a porter shaking my shoulders and asking me to follow him. I rose from the hospital trolley where I'd slept fully clothed and followed him into the main area of the emergency department. Lord Owen, the European Commission Representative in Sarajevo at the time, had arrived on an unscheduled visit to the hospital. He was surprised to see a fellow countryman within the line of white-coated medics he was addressing and asked me to brief him on the situation in the hospital. I could do no better than take him to see the shell holes in the sides of the intensive care unit. He was clearly shocked by what he'd seen and visibly moved by the sight of so many beds filled with so many bloodied and mutilated civilians. He said he was on his way to yet further negotiations with the Serbs and could now counter the claims they were making that they never fired on such targets. When I raised it myself with the UN, I was informed that the suspicion was there was a mortar placement on top of the trauma unit where I was working, and the Serbs were firing back. In war what initially appears black and white almost inevitably ends up grey. Years later, Lord Owen told me that what he saw that early morning in the hospital had a profound effect on his approach to his negotiations with the Serbs.

At midday on Saturday 5 February 1994, sixty-eight people were killed and 144 more were seriously wounded when a mortar shell exploded in the centre of a crowded marketplace in the centre of Sarajevo. I knew the marketplace well. It was enclosed between buildings on three sides, and the blast would have been both contained and concentrated in such a relatively confined space.

Who fired the mortar was a source of conjecture, as these things so often are. I received a telephone call at the trauma centre in the UK where I was on duty. I was asked to travel to Sarajevo to manage the casualties from the bombing and to report back on how best the UK government might help. By the early hours of Monday, thirty-six hours after the bombing, the team had assembled in Ancona ready to board the first UN airlift of the day into Sarajevo. The hospital I arrived at was in a state of shock. Some of the staff had been in the marketplace and survived the bombing, only to rush to the hospital to receive the injured. Others had lost friends and relatives, and all were traumatised. My notes at the time record 'it was clear that a major medical evacuation was underway. This was accepted by the doctors as the most appropriate course of action. Pride in their ability to cope, no matter what, has clearly given way to a desire for relief from a burden they have shouldered for so long.'

By the Thursday, the security situation was now extremely tense, and NATO was threatening retaliatory air strikes. Without my knowledge WHO, who had requested my team's presence in the city, precipitously withdrew their own international members from Sarajevo and back to the safety of their headquarters in Zagreb. Over a satellite telephone I spoke with London and found myself offering to stay. The civil servant on the other end of the line was studiously trying not to influence me either way, but when I told him my mind was made up, he said how useful that would be. It was in some ways a spontaneous decision, influenced by not wishing to leave colleagues in the hospital in their hour of need, and in other ways partially down to my continuing fear of the airlift. I know that the risk of dying in an all-out war with the Serbs while a NATO bombing raid was going on was greater than risk of the airlift being shot down before it all kicked off, but I had never recovered from the shooting down of the Italian airlift and the loss of those kind Italian airmen with whom I'd formed a brief friendship. Each time I flew on the airlift my dread became worse. I discussed my telephone conversation with two military paramedics who were working with us in Sarajevo – Tony Wright and Andy Shepherd – and they said they were staying as well. I felt fortunate that the UN military presence in the city at the time was now led by the UK General Sir Michael Rose, former Director of Special Forces. That evening, two members of the Special Forces knocked on the door of the apartment where I was staying. 'If the balloon goes up' they said, 'stand at the door and we will come and get you.' 'How will I know if the balloon goes up?', I asked. 'Oh, you will,' they said. 'But what if I stand here and you don't turn up?' 'Then we're all fu*ked', he said, and he left.

Just as some years before when lying in my tent on the Iran–Iraq border wondering if a missile strike was imminent, I actually slept quite well. The following morning the dawn broke over a peaceful city. The threatened airstrike was avoided and a fragile ceasefire began to emerge.

We continued working in the hospital and then once more I returned to my work in the NHS – but not for long. A week or so later, I received a call from a senior civil servant saying that there was to be an upcoming meeting between the Prime Minister John Major and the US President Bill Clinton. The outcome of this meeting, I was told, would be a 'UK/US initiative for reconstruction of essential services in Sarajevo,' and I was to start drafting now what should be the recommendations for the rehabilitation of the health system, so that we were ready to implement them when they were announced in two weeks' time. 'So that's how it works,' I thought to myself. Of course, the world's leaders don't meet for a few days and then announce a complex programme. The bulk of it is already done by their officials, and they simply ratify it (or not) when they meet. And so, the initiative was duly announced, and in March 1994, a UK–US mission was dispatched to Sarajevo to put the meat on the bones of the framework that had just been announced. Myself and my American counterpart, Dr Brent Burkholder from The Centre for Disease Control (CDC) in Atlanta, Georgia, were the medical members of a twenty-person mission. Having met with health officials in Sarajevo we finalised our recommendations. The UK government agreed to fund the health output from the UK–US mission, and I was asked to submit a proposal for its implementation. The submission was successful and so in April 1994 we launched 'Operation Phoenix: Healing the Wounds of War'. This began a two-year programme of restoring surgical services, including dentistry and eye surgery; replenishing drugs and equipment; servicing damaged or neglected medical equipment; and supporting medical and nursing education. We drew volunteers from across the UK and had special support from the British Association of Plastic, Reconstructive and Aesthetic Surgeons (BAPRAS) for our specialist reconstructive surgery teams treating those severely maimed by the war.

An important element of the recommendations from the UK–US initiative was that the health programme 'must take account of the needs of those parts of Sarajevo controlled by both Bosnian and Serbian authorities and seek where possible to avoid the establishment of parallel systems with accompanying overcapacity as a result of the partition of greater Sarajevo into the two district areas.' This meant meeting with Radovan Karadzic, a former psychiatrist and now the self-declared President of the Republic of Srpska.

Once regarded as something of a joke by those who knew him at medical school in Sarajevo, and whose teenage poetry with its 'streets running red with blood,' was openly ridiculed, was taking his revenge in adulthood by shelling the institutions where he was mocked, bringing the fantasies of his poetry to frightening reality. We travelled up the mountain to the town of Pale, a now abandoned ski resort where Karadzic had made his base. As our convoy of vehicles climbed the mountain into the snow my heart felt heavier. It was obvious that Karadzic would sooner or later end up being charged as a war criminal. I had seen for myself the bloody consequences of his actions: the shelling of civilians, the snipers firing at us as we tried to cross a road, and the utter carnage he had wreaked upon his fellow citizens. So, what was the point in going to meet him? To pamper his vanity? As we reached his 'Wolf's Lair', we all had to submit to a close body search. After that we went through an airport-style metal detector and another body search. They were taking no chances; after all, there may have been a von Stauffenberg in our midst.[10] I say it now, in full candour: I had asked myself if I should be the one to kill him. Would it be worth taking one life to save many?

We entered a large room with a long horseshoe-shaped table, at the head of which was an empty seat. The rest of us had identical chairs, with a glass of water placed on the table before us of us. We looked towards the larger, more imposing, empty seat, and waited for it to be filled. And waited. The silence was eventually broken by an aide placing a glass of orange juice on the table in front of the chair, and we waited again. Then, without warning, a posse of guards marched into the room, from which emerged the man himself, Radovan Karadzic. It was a thoroughly stage-managed, choreographed piece of political theatre: the bigger chair, the bigger drinking glass, orange juice when we had water, and the wait. He addressed us through an interpreter with words I can't remember; my mind was too occupied with why I was there, with the cameras flashing – giving him all the international recognition he craved. Flattery heaped upon him simply to get him to agree to a reconstruction of what he had destroyed. A reconstruction paid for by others and not just with their money, but with their blood. And then as we were asked to stand, I realised we were being lined up to file past him and shake his hand. This was too much. Was I to debase the memory of all those whose lives he had destroyed; abandon the values I believed had driven my work, and betray my friends, colleagues and patients suffering in the city below? And selfishly, would my future forever be dogged by a photograph of me shaking hands with a mass murderer. As we shuffled slowly around the table, like guests at a wedding queueing to shake hands with the bride and groom, the British official immediately behind me was clearly reading my thoughts as he saw me moving slower and slower. Poking me in the back and pushing me forwards, he whispered sharply 'don't flatter yourself and think it's only you.' 'We all feel the same, but it's got to be done.' And in the minute or so it took me to reach him, I'd conceded. If shaking his hand was what it took to get the aid package up and running, then so be it. I shook his hand.

Despite the risks, I tried my best to work on both sides of the divide: to be impartial, neutral and independent. I moved across checkpoints, backwards and forwards between Sarajevo and Pale, culminating in a meeting at Sarajevo Airport on 4 July 1994. The Bosnian Minister of Health at the time was Professor Beganovic. He would have preferred the meeting to be held in Sarajevo itself, but Dr Kalanic, a surgeon who had worked in Sarajevo only a couple of years before, and now the 'Minister of Health' of the Republic of Srpska, insisted it be held at the airport. Sarajevo had been divided, with a front line running through it – the Serbs on one side in 'The Republic of Srpska' and the 'Muslims' on the other. The airport, though, was mostly controlled by the UN and would not involve him or his delegation travelling through Bosnian held territory. And so, the airport it was. It was agreed beforehand that the theme of the meeting would echo the UK–US initiative and see 'no duplication of specialist medical services' and 'reciprocity of specialist medical services' between the two communities. The Serb and Bosnian officials had already said they supported these principles and had asked for me to be present at the meeting, as well as the Head of WHO in Sarajevo at the time, Stephanie Simmons.

On the morning of the meeting I met with the Bosnian delegation and the minister asked if I would chair the meeting and prepare the agenda. We were taken by military convoy to the airport, hidden in the back of an APC. The Bosnians were extremely nervous, and I can picture now the growing fear in the face of the Minister sitting opposite me in the cramped armoured vehicle; our knees bumping together as the vehicle rocked this way and that over pothole ridden roads. Professor Beganovic was risking everything to attend the meeting – not only his political reputation, but potentially his life.

We arrived on time, but the Serbs were twenty minutes late. Tensions were high and after five minutes of waiting the Bosnians threatened to leave. Their honour was not to be affronted and I knew they would seize the opportunity to abandon the meeting if they could. But they were persuaded to stay. The meeting lasted two hours. It was in fact surprisingly cordial and friendly and appeared to have been a success. It was agreed that 'Operation Phoenix' would work across the ethnic divide and put a British plastic surgery team into both sides simultaneously. To avoid both a wasteful duplication of facilities and spreading our human and physical resources too thinly, our teams would make each of the two centres specialise in different areas, e.g. facial surgery in one and hand surgery in the other. Three or four patients with these conditions would be asked to if they were prepared to travel to the other side for surgery. British doctors would work alongside local doctors in both locations which would hopefully give some reassurances to the patients. It was agreed that although this was a small start, such a gesture was important and would mark a significant step forward. The meeting began to draw to a close with a further agreement to meet again by early August at the latest, when details would be finalised, and the British teams moved into place on either side of the divide by the end of that month. At the close of the meeting it was agreed that nothing would be said to the media about the patient exchange until the project was imminent, lest it be derailed. Any public statements would be limited to: 'The meeting was a success because it had taken place. There had been agreement to explore ways of exchanging specialist medical facilities. There would be another meeting.' And that was that. Or so I thought.

At the beginning of the meeting, Dr Kalanic had presented Stephanie Simmons from WHO with a letter for William Eagleton, the then UN Special Coordinator for Sarajevo. The contents of the letter he said were private. However, when the meeting had finished, he announced he would after all reveal its contents. It was a request to Mr Eagleton to hand over the former military hospital, the 'State Hospital', in Sarajevo to the Serbs. It should be manned only by

Serbs and be only for Serbs. There should be a UN protected corridor between the Serb suburb of Grbevica and the State Hospital. Also, the medical equipment in Sarajevo should be divided between the two communities in the same way it was being suggested the country be divided. So that was the plan. The meeting had been a front. The Serb side of Sarajevo may have had the military power, but it did not have a hospital and did not have the equipment to support one either. They wanted an outpost of the Republic of Srpska in the heart of Sarajevo; a hospital only for Serbs; and Serbs only to be treated by Serbs. Medical Apartheid, and the antithesis of what we they had just agreed. The Bosnian Minister remained poker-faced and said merely he would await the views of Mr Eagleton on such matters. I was speechless. We travelled back in the APC in silence. I could hardly bear to look at the Minister, crumpled and weary on the bench seat in front of me. I remembered the doubts he had immediately before the meeting, and worried about the part I had played in bringing about such a dénouement. I hoped against hope that we could still salvage something, but worse was still to come. When Dr Kalanic returned to Pale, he announced on Serb TV that the meeting had only been about handing over the State Hospital to the Serbs and dividing the medical equipment. The Serbs had been accompanied by their own TV crew, but the Bosnians were not. However, a British TV company was making a documentary of the work of Operation Phoenix and filmed the meeting. The Serb TV film of the Bosnian Minister, Professor Beganovic, agreeing in the meeting to further talks, was edited in such a way as to suggest to the viewer that he was agreeing to transfer of the State Hospital to Serb control. When the besieged citizens of Sarajevo saw the programme there was outrage at the betrayal they believed to have been carried out by their Minister. The British film crew were able to help put the record straight by giving their film to the Bosnian authorities, but the damage was done. The minister was replaced, and my tiny infant hope was strangled at birth.

In my report to the British government on these events, I concluded:

```
My plans for any further work on the Serb side
depend on the following:

Agreement of ODA. Given the blatant flouting of the
agreements reached at the meeting, everyone shares
my extreme caution. The Serbs clearly wish to get
material aid from our project but have no intentions
of sharing specialist services with the Bosnians.
   Agreement of the new Minister of Health in
Sarajevo. I'm due to discuss this and other matters
shortly with Dr Lubjic.
   Agreement of Dr Kalanic that any further meetings
are not hijacked again to make political capital. I
am unclear how he can now convince me of this.
```

I never managed to resurrect the project on the Serb side. The Bosnians' loss of faith was absolute and irretrievable. The new Bosnian minister of health had no wish to suffer the fate of his predecessor and I received no reassurances from the Serb side. My confidence too was bruised and battered; the pain made worse by the risks I'd run in the weeks before and the efforts I'd put in to setting up the meeting.

*

A month earlier I'd arrived in Sarajevo with a team of doctors and nurses and made my way as usual, through Sierra 4 checkpoint. I drove the lead Land Rover that was marked UNHCR/ODA and got through the checkpoint without difficulty. Driving the vehicle behind me was the leader of the TV documentary team filming our work. They'd offered to assist in any way they could when working alongside the team, which was particularly appreciated when transporting team members and equipment from the airport. His vehicle was unmarked, and he was stopped and ordered out of the vehicle. I got out of my vehicle and went to his assistance while Serb militia ordered all the boxes of equipment to be taken out of both our vehicles. Through their interpreter, I explained it was medical equipment. He asked if it was for 'Muslims or Serbs?' and, truthfully at that time, I could explain it was for both sides. I was given a knife to open all the boxes. Our sleeping bags and food were allowed back in the vehicles, but all the medical equipment was ordered to be taken into the checkpoint building. I refused. I stopped a passing UN vehicle. The French officers inside spoke English and I explained the situation to them; that British medical aid was being taken. I asked for their help. The Serb police officer approached me, and through his interpreter, said I was about to be arrested. As I turned to remonstrate further with him, the French UN vehicle sped away. There was another French APC nearby whose occupants I saw were watching everything as it unfolded. They too made no move to assist.

I was escorted into the police station along with all our equipment. I explained to the police that I had a meeting already arranged in Pale for the next day. This caused a little uncertainty and I no longer seemed to be under threat of imminent arrest. He said that if Pale gave me a paper with instructions to release the equipment, I could collect it from the police station in Ilija. We drove into Sarajevo minus our equipment. Operation Phoenix was already well underway, and we were rotating surgical teams in and out of Sarajevo. The system we established, whereby outgoing teams planned the surgery for the incoming teams, was working well.

I reported what had happened to the newly appointed British ambassador in Sarajevo, and together we went to Pale and met with Dr Kalanic. Professor Staravic was also at the meeting and requested assistance from Operation Phoenix for his work in Foca. It was at that meeting that I had first discussed the movement of patients between the two communities – the plan that was put on the table at the airport meeting. My contemporaneous notes record that both Prof Staravic and Dr Kalanic said 'they would treat Muslim patients at Foca, for which they would expect to charge the Bosnian authorities' I emphasised then the importance of non-duplication of specialist medical services across the two communities and the need for reciprocity. I recorded 'this was accepted, and Dr Kalanic asked me if I would discuss these proposals further with the Bosnian authorities.' So, the opening bid was the Serbs would treat 'Muslim' patients from Sarajevo on their side but at a price (and using equipment donated by the British government). Over the coming weeks this was negotiated into an agreement to reciprocate across the ethnic divide.

Dr Kalanic apologised profusely for the seizure of the equipment and gave me his assurances that if we went to the police station in Ilija, the equipment would be returned. This I did, but the commander was not there and so we were told to return in the morning. Again I returned, but the commander refused to assist or even speak with Pale. The excuse was that he would only take his orders from the ministry of the interior and not the ministry of health.

Trying to put all this to one side, I carried on with the aid programme as best I could and went to the main hospital in Sarajevo where I met with its head, Professor Konhodjic. We discussed the proposal for joint working across the ethnic divide, to which he gave his support. On 10 June Dr Prescott, my colleague of many years, and by now working with UK-Med in Sarajevo, eventually retrieved our equipment from Ilija: in full and undamaged.

I travelled again to Pale on 15 June and met once more with Professor Staravic. My contemporaneous notes recorded 'it was accepted that the logistics and politics of treating patients in opposite communities were not to be underestimated but the need for this development at some time in the future was obvious.' Nevertheless, I was asked to convey to the Bosnian minister of health a request from the Serbs to attend a meeting of the two ministers of health to discuss these matters. Present should be the two Ministers of Health and the Heads of the Hospitals and Medical Faculties on both sides.

The meeting should attempt to reach agreement on the principles of no duplication of specialist medical services and reciprocity of specialist medical services. If such an agreement could be reached, then further discussions should take place to establish an experiment whereby Bosnian patients were treated in Foce and Serb patients treated in the University Teaching Hospital in Sarajevo. To provide reassurance to patients from both communities, international doctors would be present at both places throughout the period of the experiment. Just as was agreed at the airport meeting.

The following day the Bosnian Minister of health agreed to the principles and encouraged me to bring the two medical services together. He asked me to arrange a meeting between the two sides at the airport for the week beginning 3 July 1994. My hopes were so high, my spirits soared.

But after the airport meeting my soaring spirits crashed to earth and I felt both profoundly betrayed, but equally profoundly naïve. I berated myself about how much vanity may have played a part in my thinking I could achieve something that was eluding so many others – that I could bring these communities together. In my defence I had thought that the enlightened self-interest of securing medical care might have prevailed over sectarian and religious hatred. But not this time. I carried on working in Sarajevo, but not on the Serb side. I was not invited and was advised against it.

*

In October 1994, and seemingly out of nowhere, I received a fax message from Professor Starovic, a surgeon now working in the Republic of Srpska. I knew him. He had previously been the Dean of the Faculty of Medicine at the University of Sarajevo, and a founder of the Department of Plastic and Reconstructive Surgery at the University Medical Centre; a department once world-famous for its expertise and pioneering surgery. In his message, he reminded me of my visits to Foca earlier in the year, and of the meeting at the airport. He summarised what I knew we'd agreed at the airport, stating that each plastic surgery centre on either side of the divide would be providing specialist services for 'the whole area of the former Bosnia-Herzegovina'. I noted the reference to 'former'. He made no mention though of the request for the creation of a Serb only hospital in the centre of Sarajevo. He went on to say that although there was no written agreement between us, 'I'm accustomed to see fulfilled all promises given by my colleagues'. It was a hard message to read. He had done great work in his time.

In his obituary of 2005, published by the Faculty of Medicine in what was now called 'the University of East Sarajevo' in Foca, he was described as facing an assassination attempt on 6 April 1992 – first day of the war. 'He spent 400 days as prisoner at the clinic which has been (sic) founded and led by him twenty years. After leaving Sarajevo, he became the Dean of the Faculty of Medicine, University of Sarajevo, Republic of Srpska.' I know that the plastic surgery department in Sarajevo was predominantly a Serb led institution, and I could never resolve clearly whether the Serb plastic surgeons were forced out, left of their own accord, or left reluctantly for their own safety. Whatever, I always felt that Professor Starovic had lost a great deal; and that he knew it. His email darkened in tone. 'Having deep trust in you, I was exposed to some rather unpleasant questions asked by my eminent fellow doctor, surgeons and university professors: 'have Doctor Tony Redmond and your friends aligned with the Muslim side? ... Has politics interfered with the Phoenix programme or has it made British plastic surgeons change their minds?' The message concluded 'therefore I find your failure to keep your promises strange and unacceptable. I feel very upset knowing that the programme has been in the process (sic.) in the Muslim part of Sarajevo for the last three months.' Although addressed to me personally, it ended '... regardless of all political connotations and British government's relations to this part of the former Bosnia-Herzegovina. Looking forward to receiving your answer, which you may fax to the Ministry of health Dragan Kalanic or to the fax in Belgrade (Serbia).'

That fax was dated 10 October 1994. A little over two weeks later, a UNHCR convoy carrying ten aircraft pallets of mixed WHO and UK-Med medical supplies and equipment was stopped at a Serb-controlled checkpoint en route from the airport to the city. The UN drivers were ordered to take the trucks to a nearby Serbian warehouse where everything was removed. Almost twelve hours later the drivers were ordered to return empty-handed to Sarajevo. Shortly afterwards, with colleagues from WHO, I once again travelled to Pale and met with Dr Kalinic. He apologised, particularly for taking the WHO medical supplies, with the unconvincing excuse that the paperwork had been incorrect. That checkpoint, Sierra 4, was the one we all used regularly. His claim it was a mistake was weakened by his simultaneous demand for 50 per cent of the UK-Med supplies they held. I realised I was now moving into politics and no longer acting entirely independently. The confiscated equipment had been entirely funded by the British government, a representative of which gave me some handwritten briefing notes prior to this meeting. I was to give absolutely no guarantees but to look at what they needed rather than agree to a blanket share of everything that might include things they might have no use for, but I was to make no promises. I was to say that we would not work on the Serb side to release the confiscated equipment – there was to be no linkage between the two. Once the equipment was returned though, we could move on and look to applying the established UN (23 per cent Serb/77 per cent Bosnian) split of future equipment, but there must be no other preconditions to its release.

We never got the equipment back.

7.

Abandoned Babies

Kosovo

After four years of moving frantically between clinical work in the NHS, academic work in the University, and continuous humanitarian missions into the war-torn former Yugoslavia, I was exhausted; both physically and emotionally. I had also begun experiencing several worrying symptoms that I knew should be investigated. But there was always another mission, something that I really must do.

In June 1999 I took a call from Dr Mukesh Kapila, no longer of the Overseas Development Administration (ODA), but now the Head of the Conflict and Humanitarian Affairs Department of the new Department for International Development (DFID). Direct as ever, he asked if I would lead a medical assessment mission to the clinical centre in Pristina in the Serbian region of Kosovo. The war in the Balkans had moved on from Bosnia, and following their bombing of Belgrade, NATO had moved its troops from Macedonia up into Kosovo.

It had become increasingly clear to me towards the end of my work in Sarajevo that I really was not well, and with my work in the Balkans now complete, I faced up to seeing my GP. Throughout 1997 I faced a succession of consultations, investigations and surgical operations. After each I kept returning to work, but I was becoming progressively weaker and losing weight. In 1998 it was recommended to me by the hospital occupational health department that I retire from my consultant post in the NHS on the grounds of ill health. I refused. Being a doctor was an integral part of my identity and I couldn't bear to just stop at forty-seven. A kind and perceptive human resources manager, Sally Campbell, saw my anguish and understood my refusal to let go. She spoke to me at length and reassured me that this was not the end of my career. I was only pressing the pause button. It was an opportunity to get well and resume my career later. I owe her a lot. She gave me a story to tell myself; a mantra to recite. I was only stepping back until my health was better.

Eventually my health improved enough to allow me to start some part time medical advisory work. That was when I took the call from Mukesh. The brief was to lead a health scoping mission to the University Clinical Centre in Pristina, Kosovo, for a month in June and July. I felt fit enough to take on a short, if somewhat risky, mission to Kosovo. My GP agreed. As it turned out, it was riskier than I thought and much longer than I'd planned. I was ultimately away for a year.

Mukesh Kapila and his colleague, Rob Holden, had entered Kosovo alongside NATO. They found the Clinical Centre in Pristina to be highly volatile, in a poor state of repair and inadequately equipped. The head of the hospital, a Serb, was struggling to maintain control over a hospital that was now under siege from several thousand returning Albanians, claiming, or reclaiming as they would say, the hospital as their own. Old resentments erupted everywhere into acts of violence. They had heard gunfire in the surgical emergency room at the time of their visit. The head of surgery, like the head of all the clinics during the preceding ten years, had also been a Serb, and was now missing. When I was later to become the head of the hospital, I received daily calls from his wife, now in Belgrade, begging me to tell her of his whereabouts. That is, until we were all forced to accept he had been murdered by Albanians.

We left by air for Skopje, then travelled overland through Macedonia, crossed the border into Kosovo, and continued up towards Pristina. On my arrival at the Clinical Centre I was met by Lt Colonel (later Major General) Jeremy Rowan. In the immediate aftermath of the NATO invasion, the British Army had seized control of the clinical centre, which was now under his command. Jeremy briefed the team and arranged meetings with key players in the hospital, including Dr Illir Tolaj, with whom I would forge a lasting friendship. I would learn later from Illir that three years previously his father, while sitting as a high court judge, had been shot dead in open court by a Serb. Illir himself had worked for the Red Cross and was severely injured the year before when his Red Cross vehicle entered a minefield. Later, talking long into the night, Illir was to open up to me about how he and his companion, Dr. Sheptim Robaj, were blown out of the vehicle and lay side-by-side in the minefield, both too injured to move. Sheptim, who was also his closest friend, was an anaesthetist. As they lay there together waiting for help, it became clear to the two doctors that Sheptim had suffered severe internal injuries from which he was now bleeding uncontrollably. Illir held him in his arms as his friend made him memorise his dying message to his wife and children and promise him that he would relay it, verbatim, should Illir survive. His friend died in his arms. Illir survived, despite suffering a broken back, and kept his promise. He was eventually evacuated to Switzerland for treatment and on recovery he returned to Kosovo, to continue his medical work. For all he had suffered and all the threats he would continue to endure, I never saw Illir in anything but a kind and good humour. An exceptional doctor doing his best for, and seeing the best in, others.

The team was quickly able to assess the immediate needs of the hospital and reported these back to DFID in London. We saw for ourselves the fragility and instability that Mukesh had described, as more Albanian staff returned to the hospital and Serbs felt increasingly threatened. A Bulgarian UN worker on his first day in Pristina was shot dead in the street simply for asking him the time. He'd spoken in Serbian to an Albanian. An elderly Serb woman shuffled along the hallway to her flat to answer the knocking at her front door. She was murdered in a hail of bullets fired though the door as she began to turn the lock. Serbs were leaving in ever increasing numbers. Albanians, now reversing the ethnic cleansing they had suffered so terribly, set about what seemed to me like an endless round of revenge killings. Within a matter of days, the Serb majority in the hospital had been replaced by a large and expanding Albanian majority. Every day more people arrived at the hospital claiming that they worked there before they were expelled by the Serbs, or they should work there now the Serbs had gone. We had no way of knowing if their claims were true. Most troubling was that we had no way of knowing if they were medically qualified. Many were not, in the traditional sense.

Prior to 1990, Kosovo enjoyed a great deal of autonomy within the former Yugoslavia. However, in 1989, the Serb regime, under Slobodan Milosevic, had begun a process of removing Albanians from positions of authority. I understand this was a political move to rekindle ethnic tensions and so bolster support for a resurgence of Serb nationalism. Not long after this, in 1992, when I was in Kosovo inspecting medical facilities as part of my work for WHO, I was taken to Kosovo Polje by my Serb 'minder' to see a monument there to the war dead. I was very moved as he stood, head bowed, hands clasped in front of him, tears slowly running down his face; a solitary figure in the windswept desolate 'Field of Crows'. I knew little of Balkans history then, and assumed this was a monument to some recent, perhaps even the current, conflict. It was in fact a monument to a battle in 1389 when the Serbs were defeated by the Turks of the Ottoman Empire. If I needed any demonstration of just how much this new Serb nationalism had mythologised this defeat, here it was: a grown man weeping before a stranger, for the dead of a battle fought 600 years ago. By casting the predominantly Muslim Albanians as the torch bearers of the Ottomans, and braying for the righting of the perceived wrongs of centuries, it was but a frighteningly short step sideways into the ethnic cleansing that was to follow.

On that first visit to Kosovo, the Serb doctors who were now, not altogether voluntarily, relocated from Belgrade, told me that the Albanians had insisted that teaching in the medical school must be in Albanian. When this was refused, they walked out; or according to the Albanians, were expelled. They set up an unofficial and, under Serb law, illegal, underground health system; the so-called 'parallel health system.' This comprised private clinics in doctors' homes, including surgical operating theatres, and clinics run by the Mother Theresa humanitarian organisation. At least the founders of this parallel system had been trained in the internationally recognised Yugoslav system. The real concern for us lay with the parallel medical school they'd also set up. How students gained admission to this I could never determine exactly, but by 1999 two cohorts of medical and dental students had received their training in this clan-destine, makeshift, and unlicensed system. The Albanian community accepted them as qualified doctors, but from what I could judge they had very limited clinical experience. Even they acknowledged it.

Crowded into the now vacated medical director's office, the team met with a large group of Albanian doctors, WHO and Serb representatives, where with much shouting and jockeying for position, the Albanians were demanding to take control of the hospital. Not surprisingly, this was rejected vigorously by the Serbs, even though Albanians were already occupying much of the building. As a way forwards, we proposed to the room a 'hospital management board' should be established, with representation from all the disparate groups. This was eventually accepted but there followed yet more argument, this time between the Albanians themselves as to which of them (it would never be a Serb) would chair the board and so lead the hospital. To break this final deadlock, we suggested there be an international appoint-ment as the temporary head of the hospital, and with Jeremy's help and the connections he had already established, I was accepted as the Medical Director for a three-month term of office. We subse-quently appointed international advisors to support each specialty: a director of finance and a facilities manager. Dr Simonovic, Deputy Minister of Health, also in the room, accepted and approved my appointment and this approach was endorsed and ratified by the UN.

WHO, out of expediency I guess, quickly decided that qualifica-tions gained in the parallel system should be recognised and, surprisingly, so did Dr Simonovic. But he did push for equal numbers of Serbs and Albanians on the board and it was the aim of the international team to make the board as representative as possible. As per tradition, heads of clinics were voted in by the senior doctors in that specialty. However, there were complaints that voting was not free and fair. We 'took soundings' on the political background of candidates and drew up what we thought to be a reasonably representative board. However, this did not meet with the approval of the 'temporary government' of Hashim Thaci who had now appointed his own parallel Ministry of Health. Thaci had been a leader of the Kosovo Liberation Army (KLA) and his reputation amongst my Albanian colleagues at the time was fearsome. He subsequently became Prime Minister and was until recently President of Kosovo. At the time of writing he was awaiting the outcome at the Hague of indictments for war crimes, crimes against humanity, murder, enforced disappearance, persecution and torture.

One morning I received a rather threatening visitation from this parallel ministry. Without any formalities as I recall, I was informed by a somewhat burly individual that the ministry, i.e. Thaci, had drawn up their own hospital board, with its own head. A paper was placed upon my desk on which there was a list of names. I carefully pointed out that there were other points of view to be considered but thanked him for the advice and I promised to get back to Mr Thaci. I discussed the situation with colleagues, and to avoid unnecessary conflict, but most of all to avoid the hospital splitting into two factions, I proposed a compromise whereby the ministry's board was incorporated into that already proposed by me. My rationale for compromise was reinforced by the recent experience of the international head of the hospital in Peja, in the Serb enclave of Kosovo, who having failed to reach a compromise, found himself completely side-lined by internal differences to such a degree that the hospital's own self-appointed board met independently outside of the hospital. I was determined to try to avoid a new 'parallel system' being allowed to develop and my compromise solution was ultimately accepted. In practice, many of the appointees appeared on both lists anyway, and where there was a potential conflict, we appointed each to the board. But I also added UN observers from WHO, OSCE and UNHCR to demonstrate and ensure public accountability. The board, I insisted, was also to be multi-ethnic. Whilst candidates proposed by the temporary ministry of health were all Albanian, and basically KLA activists, I also added two Serb paediatricians, a Montenegrin Muslim, and a Turk to the board. They received threats to their lives. I offered them protection within the hospital, but these threats were largely made outside, which is where they felt lay the greatest threat. Within a matter of weeks, they left. The board, and indeed the hospital, became solely Albanian.

Or so I thought. One Serb doctor stayed throughout. She was a Serb married (now widowed) to an Albanian and in her sixties. She never left her post and no one ever complained about her or threatened her. There were also a handful of Serb nurses and pharmacists – exact numbers were difficult for me to establish without drawing dangerous attention to their presence. There were also small signs of encouragement. One Serb nurse was threatened by a female Albanian hospital security guard and told to leave. We suspended the guard and interviewed the nurse. The army offered to escort her to Serbia. However, when she found out that the woman who threatened her did so because her husband had been killed in the war, she said it was bad enough to lose your husband – she shouldn't lose her job as well. The Albanian nurses on her ward offered to protect her, and she stayed.

One of the saddest conversations I had was with the young medical and dental students. They had been in the parallel system for half their lives and were bursting to explode onto a broader European stage. They were also confused, and I sensed perhaps a little disappointed, by my persistent efforts to integrate non-Albanians into the hospital. I said that the ultimate effect of their approach would be a mono-ethnic society, anathema to the Europe they so desperately wanted to join. 'That's right,' they said. 'We'll be the first.'

I nevertheless held regular meetings with the Serb community and two Serb doctors once asked to return to their posts. The moderate doctors in the hospital took the view that 'as long as they don't have blood on their hands,' they could return. But there was deep concern that many Serb doctors colluded with the security forces. Albanians said they found secret police files in doctors' offices though I saw no evidence of this. These two doctors were viewed as good colleagues, I discovered, and deemed to be innocent of any crimes. The Albanian doctors said they would be welcomed back without a problem and the army investigated their security en route to and from the hospital. The UNHCR, however, cautioned against them returning, saying that no one could guarantee their safety, and an incident would be dangerously destabilising (their words). So, they never returned.

One cannot overemphasise the fragility of the hospital in those early weeks and months. The euphoria of the Albanian reclamation of the hospital was quickly replaced by disappointment and inertia. The energies of rebellion were quickly being turned against the international community in the face of the realities of peace. The hospital clearly needed a massive investment and the staff were increasingly reminded of the professional penalty they had paid for their years of exclusion. While their aspirations for the future immediately after NATO may have been wildly unrealistic, even the most down-to-earth had not expected they would have to work in the public sector for nothing. Failure by UNMIK (the United Nations Mission in Kosovo) to pay public sector salaries was the greatest threat to public order and social stability in the immediate post-war phase. Our efforts were severely compromised by the loss of faith the Albanians felt in a UN administration that expected them to work for nothing, compounded by the high salaries the UN were paying local people to work for them. After an initially hostile response and protracted negotiations, UNMIK finally allowed us to use a grant from DFID to commence the payment of stipends.

Once agreed, Arthur Pittman, our international director of finance, drew up a list of all our registered employees and announced a schedule for the payments. There were no banks operating so a large amount of cash had been brought overland from Macedonia and secured in a heavy safe, in a guarded room, ready for distribution the next day. In the early hours I was awoken by a call from the UN police to tell me the room had been broken into and the impossibly heavy safe taken. The guard had seen and heard nothing. I couldn't blame the guard for his temporary loss of faculties. Kosovo is a very small, and then very dangerous, place, and the safety of his family was uppermost in his mind. I had a pretty good idea who was behind it – as did everyone else. Having pressed so hard to get the money it was heart-breaking to see it taken. Such was the importance to the stability of the hospital of paying the staff at least something, the British government, who had supplied the funds originally, was persuaded to give it another shot. This time there would be no announcements. When the money arrived, it was to be distributed immediately. The system for getting the money into Pristina was like something out of a spy movie. Members of the British aid team had regular trips to the airport in Skopje, Macedonia to pick up staff and goods. On each trip you were now told the code word for the day, and if someone tapped you on the shoulder at the airport, you were to take the hold-all they were carrying. No matter what you thought you were there to do, you went back to your vehicle, and with the bag under your seat, drove directly to the hospital. It happened to me once.

When I took over as head of the hospital, there was an armed paratrooper placed at the door of my office. There was an armoured vehicle in the hospital grounds. We would never be a normal hospital in such circumstances, I judged, so I asked for them to be removed. I was warned in no uncertain terms of the risks in general, and to me in particular, though I thought privately this exaggerated my true value as a target. The uplifting effect on hospital morale was immediate, and tangible with every hand that shook mine.

This need to look and act like a normal hospital extended for me to a patient's rights to privacy. The world's media were roaming the hospital at the start. 'VIPs' would visit the hospital, unannounced, and proceed to clinical departments without a thought that they should seek permission – something unthinkable elsewhere in Europe. NGOs and even UN organisations, would turn up with cameras and VIPs, without notice or permission, and wander around the hospital. This badly undermined our efforts to demonstrate to local people that the hospital was theirs and normality was returning. Worse still, these VIPs and the media seemed obsessed with mutilated children. Children with limbs missing from landmine explosions and disfiguring injuries from cluster bombs. We tried hard to explain how detrimental it was to their recovery if they only ever received attention whilst they appeared to be mutilated. How they were less likely to adopt their artificial limbs and return to some degree of normality if they perceived that by so doing, they would lose the attention they craved. Several times we cradled injured children who, having performed for the world's cameras and VIPs, broke down in tears when they'd left.

An early rumour circulating amongst the international community was that there were 'abandoned babies' in the paediatric unit. The press wanted to photograph them, and a military officer wanted to take one home with him to America. He turned up in my office saying he was due to go home the following day, knew of the abandoned babies, and was here to take one home with him. I explained that it was yet to be confirmed they were truly abandoned. UNICEF, as the approved officials in such circumstances, were tracing relatives and only if none were identified after at least three months would formal Kosovar adoption procedures be initiated. On arrival in country UNICEF found twenty-four 'abandoned' children in the paediatric ward. Because of the conflict, social services had been unable to facilitate foster care or adoption during the previous two years. They had been left for many hours tied into their cots, with severe developmental delay the result. UNICEF quickly set about improving their care, installing a playroom into the paediatric ward, and designating 'substitute mothers' to give them each the touch, care, and attention they so badly needed. Six of these children were reunited with their parents, fifteen placed in foster care and two successfully adopted. A small number of children continued to be 'abandoned' in the hospital, but they were well looked after and the process of fostering and adoption satisfactorily established.

I warned the soldier too of the complexities of international adoption. He was astounded. He couldn't accept or believe a 'country such as this' would have any formal adoption procedures, and in any event he was offering a poor child the opportunity of a Christian upbringing in America which I was wrong to deny. He became angry and belligerent as I patiently and repeatedly explained the legalities, but in the end, I had to say very firmly that I would not allow him, or anyone else, to walk in here and take a baby, abandoned or otherwise, anywhere. His final gambit was that he'd already promised a baby to his sister in the states and couldn't go home tomorrow without one. I asked him to leave, which he did without good grace and with much complaint. I escorted him to the door of the hospital, saw him leave the grounds, then put guards on the paediatric unit.

So-called 'abandoned' babies were not new to me. As a young doctor in Salford, UK, I was struggling to convince the parents of what looked to me like a very healthy child that he didn't need to come into hospital. That is until the more experienced night sister pulled me to one side and explained. It was Christmas Eve, this was a poor family, and every year they brought the youngest of their children to A&E with a similar story of fictitious illness. 'Just admit the wee mite,' she said, 'They know he will be safe here, get a Christmas dinner, and a visit from Father Christmas with presents they couldn't afford.' She assured me they would pick him up in a few days' time, and so they did. It was the same in Kosovo. Some children were orphaned and left in the hospital when their parents were killed in the war, but others were deposited with us until their parents considered it safe enough to reclaim them. In these international emergencies, it is the role of UNICEF to safeguard these children, a job they do well, and over the time I was there, most, but sadly not all, of the 'abandoned babies' were reunited with relatives or safely adopted within Kosovo.

The double standards of 'doing good' to poorer countries in ways you would consider inconceivable, and morally wrong, at home extended to the famous. Actresses arrived unannounced, and the owner of a well-known cosmetics company made an unauthorised visit and refused to consult with any of the management team when confronted. We found their beauty products in the pharmacy, with labels only in English. The potential for their misuse was obvious and they were removed. A UNICEF goodwill ambassador did ask for permission to visit the children's ward but cancelled at the last minute. Their press office confirmed to me this was because we had asked them not to film the injured children. It was left to me to tell the children, all washed and spruced up for the visit, that it wouldn't now go ahead.

The hospital board functioned fairly well – better than expected, in many ways. But there were disruptive elements, particularly in surgery. Surgical procedures tend to fetch the highest bounty in a 'cash for operations culture', so the stakes are high. He (and in Kosovo then it would only ever be a he) who controlled surgery could monopolise a great deal of wealth and power. At the core of this and wider disruption in the hospital was the continued presence, and threat, of the KLA. It seemed to me that any success within the hospital that could be attributed to the international community threatened the perceived dependency of the local people on the KLA for their protection and future prosperity. I say this because most, and perhaps all, the dissidents on the board were (ex-) KLA. The additional factor, and no country is immune to this, was that the surgeons continuing private income (which was substantial) was dependent on the public perception that the hospital could not meet their needs.

I felt I needed to meet with Mr Thaci, and Dr Tolaj arranged a meeting at which he translated. I described the disruption in the hospital: staff not turning up for work, the threats and instability. I told him that however long I stayed at the hospital, it would only ever be temporary. I felt sure that if he used his influence then things could settle down, and for a time the hospital improve; the benefits of which would be there for his taking when I left. He reacted furiously, demanding to know why I should think any if this had anything to do with him. The meeting ended abruptly, and I left downcast and now very much afraid. The next morning, the doorman, who had left his post some time back, was back at work and greeted me with a smile. The hospital was alive and working: floors were being cleaned, rubbish being cleared. I was sitting bewildered in my office when the same henchman who had delivered to me Thaci's list of board members, popped his head round the door and with a grin and thumbs up said 'Mr Thaci say everything OK now?'

If things settled down within the hospital, they didn't outside. I was reminded of this every time I met with the new Albanian co-director of health and social welfare and saw a pistol he barely hid tucked unholstered into his waist band. I was reminded even more starkly when I picked up the phone on my desk and heard a voice shouting 'Come quickly. Come to the operating Room. A patient is threatening to explode a grenade!' I broke the few seconds of my shocked silence with a nervous request for more details.

Another elderly Serb lady had been shot multiple times while walking in the street. She had been brought to us by ambulance, still alive, just about talking, but bleeding heavily from the wounds within her abdomen. As I left my office, I gave instructions to alert the British Army, and made my way to the scene. I was met in the corridor outside of the operating theatre by a group of hospital staff surrounding an elderly lady lying curled up on a hospital trolley. The lady was holding something metallic in the tight grip of both her hands: a hand grenade. And here was the dilemma. She needed urgent lifesaving surgery. She believed that as the hospital was now in the grip of the Albanians and it was Albanians who had just shot her, then they would simply finish the job off were she to submit to surgery here in Pristina. She wanted to be transferred to the safety of Belgrade. But she was so badly wounded and bleeding so heavily, she would die before we could complete the journey. She threatened to detonate the grenade if we did not comply. As she continued to bleed out before us, she was destined to lapse into unconsciousness, when she would also gradually lose her grip on the grenade. Could we judge the exact moment when it was safest to snatch the grenade? We couldn't wait too long to decide, I figured, as by the time she bled out to the point of unresponsiveness – the point up to where her life might be possibly be saved would likely have passed. So, we needed to intervene, both in her best interests and for the safety of those who were crowded around her and her ticking time bomb. We rapidly agreed a plan that would acknowledge her fears, respect her wishes as best we could, and bring the crisis to a close. I asked the anaesthetist to sedate her while the army personnel were poised ready to seize the grenade as soon as she appeared to become drowsy. She would then be whisked into the operating theatre where a British Army surgeon and a Lebanese surgeon working with MDM Greece would carry out damage limitation surgery to stem the bleeding. The British Army would then transfer her rapidly to Belgrade, where definitive surgery would be completed. She might go off to sleep in Pristina, but she would wake up in Belgrade as she had wished. We were all set to go. Then a voice from the back said softly, but very firmly; 'She hasn't given her consent. You cannot intervene. It is against her human rights.' Everyone stopped dead. They turned to her, then to me. I looked towards the voice, and recognised it as coming from a young doctor: a volunteer from North America. Time, having appeared to momentarily stand still, now picked up speed as all of us realised that without a decision of some sort very soon, events would unfold of their own disastrous accord. I addressed the small group around the patient and said 'As Medical Director of the Hospital I take full responsibility and my instructions are to put her to sleep now, as planned, take her into theatre and stop the bleeding, then transfer her to Belgrade.' Without hesitation the team leapt into action. Drugs were administered, her eyes closed, the Army took the grenade from her and she disappeared into the operating theatre. An hour or so later she was in an ambulance speeding through Kosovo with a military escort and woke up between the crisp sheets of a hospital bed in Belgrade from where she would go on to make a full recovery.

I made my way back to my office where I sat in my chair and laid my head on the desk in sheer exhaustion and relief. But not for long. My assistant came in and said that the North American doctor was here and wanted to see me; urgently. I looked at her pleadingly, hoping she would put her off. I've tried to say you are busy she said, but she is in no mood to take no for an answer. I straightened myself out and asked her to show her in. So, this is my 'Waterloo', I thought. My bridge too far. One too many chances taken. She was here to tell me that she would report me and who knew what would follow?

She came in and sat in front of my desk. 'I am so sorry,' she said. 'I don't know what I was thinking. I was caught up in the moment and couldn't grasp the enormity of the situation. I've come to apologise.'

I told her that she did what she thought was right and had spoken up for the patient. It had worked out well in the end. We parted and stayed as friends. She carried on doing great work in the hospital and went on from there to a successful and laudable career in humanitarian medicine.

*

Looking back now, and given the uncertainties that remain in and around Kosovo, I sometimes wonder what we achieved. Although the familiar sequence of early liberators morphing into occupiers unfolded over time, it was not before we handed over the reins to the local (now wholly Albanian) medical community and my role became more advisory than managerial. Importantly, the hospital stayed open and functioning, and is still open now. Moreover, it improved and developed. I confirmed as much when I visited again a few years ago. We exposed the isolated Albanian doctors to modern medical practice and introduced to the hospital more accountability with audit, formal medical note keeping, and the basic tenets of good medical practice such as written consent for surgical operations. All absent when we arrived. When I first arrived I'd been called to a surgical meeting where the professor of surgery was threatening to shoot the professor of pathology. 'Why?' I asked. 'He called me a liar,' said the Professor of Surgery. 'Did you?' I asked the pathologist. He said that when he'd examined the appendix the surgeon had taken out from a patient he thought had appendicitis, he'd found it to be normal. 'See, I told you,' barked the surgeon. 'That's not quite what he's saying.' I suggested. 'And anyway, surely it's not enough to shoot him?' He looked me straight in the eye, and without flinching said, 'in Kosovo it is.'

In my desk I found handwritten figures collated by one of my predecessors that recorded the infant mortality and maternal mortality rates in 1990 as many times higher than elsewhere in Europe. Worse still, these earlier figures revealed that that most illness in women of childbearing years in Kosovo was due to complications of pregnancy, childbirth, and the period immediately after birth. I was not surprised. The delivery suite had been run-down and neglected. The delivery beds were old, in a terrible state of repair, and very basic. Moreover, I learned that the gynaecologists considered it a failure of their art if they had to resort to caesarean section, and women likewise thought they had failed as a woman if they could not deliver normally. This combination led to mothers labouring too long, bleeding heavily, and too many of them and their babies dying. While the rest of Europe had growing concerns about the rising numbers of Caesarean Sections, I was worried that we were doing too few. We tried our best to influence these cultural practices, but I read in the international and Kosovar press of continuing concerns over maternal mortality and a worrying failure to publish accurate data.

On our arrival there were several poorly equipped and underperforming 'intensive care' units in the hospital. Most did not have patients on life support machines. 'Intensive care' was in fact what in the rest of Europe would be considered an acute ward. In Kosovo many of the patients in the general wards were hardly ill at all. They were waiting for, or recovering from, relatively minor operations, or were unofficially paying to occupy a bed longer than was required because of the dangers outside. However, in the department of surgery, the intensive care unit had some very sick patients, usually the victims of trauma. The initial concerns about a deluge of landmine victims proved to some extent to have been unfounded, but instead there were very large numbers of road traffic accident victims, particularly children. The lack of effective intensive care was reflected in a mortality rate of over 90 per cent for ventilated patients. The combination of the new emergency centre that we built, improvements in the training of anaesthetists that we introduced and the provision of appropriate equipment in improved facilities, resulted in the mortality rate dropping to less than 40 per cent – not too far off from European norms at that time. A similar impact was achieved in neonatology. Such was the lack of skill and experience, when we first arrived, the mortality rate for ventilated babies was 100 per cent. That is every baby, regardless of birth weight, needing to be put on a life support machine, died. With the input of specialist support and training, the mortality rate in the neonatal intensive care unit quickly fell to around 40 per cent: not great but certainly better.

In addition, we encouraged and supported the return to academic life and funded the re-launch of a Kosovar medical journal called 'Praxis Medica'. And surprisingly, we found ourselves amongst the pioneers of telemedicine with the gift of what was then the cutting-edge technology of a digital camera, which we connected to a satellite phone. In one case an Albanian soldier with multiple gunshot wounds to the abdomen needed extensive life-saving surgery. His wounds had been inappropriately closed by inexperienced surgeons and he now had multiple openings in his abdomen through which faeces leaked continuously. He was septic and desperately ill. I rang a colleague in Manchester, Mr Nigel Scott, a specialist fistula surgeon, who agreed to guide the surgical team through what would be a highly complex surgical procedure. This he did from his office in Manchester, step by step, photo by photo, until all the infection had been cleared, all the dead bowel cut away, and he was left with a clean but now fully open, abdomen. Closing this complex wound was beyond the skills and facilities in

Kosovo, even with telemedicine support, but we were able to arrange his transfer to Manchester, where the wound was closed successfully, and he went on to make a full recovery. And also, to claim asylum.

We worked very closely with the International Organisation for Migration (IOM) in establishing a system for the medical evacuation of patients (MEDEVAC). I knew from my earlier work in Sarajevo just how difficult and open to abuse this could be. There, everyone wanted to be evacuated – sick and well alike – so choosing who could go was a pernicious task. The UN drew up a list of eligible and ineligible conditions. I resisted this and preferred to identify priorities: not if you go, but who should go first. We drew up similar guidelines in Kosovo and established a weekly MEDEVAC committee that included the IOM, WHO, the Dean of the Medical School and other internationals.

Inclusion on the list did not of course guarantee MEDEVAC. Far from it. The IOM had funding for transport to and from the host country and would arrange all the paperwork. However, they had to find a country willing to accept the patient and their relatives, and willing to foot the bill in its entirety. Despite these odds, the IOM did well, and by the time I left, over one third of patients listed for MEDEVAC had successfully received their treatment overseas. Just as in Sarajevo, the easiest to MEDEVAC were children with wounds to their limbs, or babies with congenital heart disease. And just as in Sarajevo, the most difficult to place were the non-photogenic adults. Worse still the elderly, and impossible were the severely mentally ill.

I tried my best but I made mistakes. Not entirely unsurprisingly, as an outsider, I never fully won over all the senior medical staff in the hospital, and as my three months term of office was extended to six months and then to twelve, those early pockets of resentment grew. And not just within the usual suspects or the Albanian Ministry. Once again, I was caught between the conflicting aims of the FCO and DFID. An invitation to a cosy fireside talk by a senior FCO official was but a thinly veiled direction to let the KLA have their way and allow matters to take their course. I didn't, and persevered, looking ahead to what was still to be done to improve patient care, and leaving my back widely exposed.

The hospital was by no means perfect, but day by day it got cleaner. Rubbish was moved, the grass was cut, and the snow was cleared. Most importantly, patients received better and better treatment. But I had made enemies and overstayed my welcome. A senior doctor who we removed from the board because of his misuse of private practice within the hospital, exacted his revenge. With the help of others, both inside and outside of the hospital, who were also looking to settle scores or destabilise our work to accelerate our exit, he facilitated a clandestine, unauthorised and highly selective tour of the hospital by a journalist, and while I was in the UK at my mother-in-law's funeral. Shall I say the article in a British Sunday newspaper that followed was not entirely flattering. It wasn't a death blow to the programme, but it highlighted our vulnerability to political shenanigans (both Kosovar and, I believe, UK), and that we were there on sufferance. I wrote a letter to the editor emphasising what I believed to have been a significant misrepresentation, but it was never acknowledged, let alone published. A BBC team who were reporting on the hospital at the same time also protested to the newspaper about misrepresentation, but also to no avail.

I made other mistakes. On our arrival there were parts of the hospital still unoccupied. One of these was the Serb administration building. We were approached by the Carabinieri, now posted to Kosovo, who offered to pay rent, supply medicines, patrol the grounds and place their doctor at the disposal of the hospital in exchange for their use of the building. It seemed a good deal and, despite reservations, I gained a general agreement to proceed. They moved in and began to renovate the building but then reneged on almost all their other promises. There were issues which I should have foreseen concerning who owned the building in those early uncertain days, and so who could claim the rent, but pleas for payment in kind were ignored. Discontent within the hospital grew and became worse when shortly after they'd occupied the building, a delegation of parents came to tell me that it had been built as a unit for disabled children, with funds raised by the local community. The Serbs had expelled the children and used the building for administration, but now the parents wanted it back. It was imperative that the Carabinieri should make good on their promises or give the building back. Yet the UN supported the Carabinieri. I even served notice on them which they ignored, and the UN still refused to intervene. I complained vigorously and tirelessly, until they eventually paid something to the hospital for the use of the premises, but they never left, and the affair undermined our role in the hospital.

*

In addition to facing up to the aftermath of a cruel and bloody war, almost eleven years after Lockerbie, I found myself once again dealing with the aftermath of another terrible plane crash. In November 1999, a plane chartered by the UN World Food Programme inbound from Rome, crashed into the mountainside in northern Kosovo. In total twenty-one UN workers and three crew members perished. No one survived. The UN had no major incident plan and tensions between different groups and nations came quickly to the surface in its aftermath. Once retrieved from the hillside, the bodies were taken to the clinical centre in Pristina, where they then came under my care. This is my contemporaneous report on the incident, which I include in full:

As you are aware the WFP plane crashed just after noon on Friday 12/11/99. There were initially conflicting messages and at one point the BBC stated the plane had arrived safely in Tirana. Ultimately the crash and the fact that there were no survivors were confirmed that evening. On the day of the crash no message was received at the hospital. Nevertheless, when it was confirmed to me by DFID, I informed the mortuary technicians of the possible reception of 24 bodies. I also went to KFOR headquarters and enquired if the bodies might be coming to the Hospital. I was told no decision had been made. Their first thought was Mitrovica hospital. I suggested they might liaise with Ljpian. They took my numbers and agreed they would make contact if it appeared the hospital in Pristina might be the best option.

Next morning, Saturday 13/11/99, two KFOR officers arrived at the hospital and informed me a container was being delivered to the hospital to store the bodies when they arrived by helicopter later that day. (This had been decided at a KFOR meeting that morning). It was to be placed in the Carabinieri car

park. I informed them the car park was some
considerable distance from the mortuary and that
the container should be placed next to the mortuary.
This was done.

A US army mass graves team was tasked by KFOR to
assist in the reception and preparation of the
bodies. We prepared an autopsy room for this
purpose. Two Albanian pathologists made themselves
available in the hospital. There was some initial
uncertainty as to whether full autopsies would be
required at this initial stage particularly on the
flight crew. The Albanian pathologists were ready to
assist in this if required.

Mr Enrique Aguilar, UNMIK Regional Administrator
Pristina, came to the hospital. He was concerned
about death certificates. We agreed that formal
certificates could not be issued until identification
and autopsies were complete. This might take some
time and be completed in another country. However,
some official documentation to record their
reception into the hospital and the fact that coffins
contained human remains would be required if the
bodies were to be moved out of the country. Mr
Aguilar and I agreed that a joint 'medical
certificate of death' signed by him as regional
administrator and myself as medical director would
be the most appropriate and this was approved by
UNMIK lawyers. These documents were later accepted
without problem by the Italian authorities when the
bodies were moved.[11]

Another issue was pressure to view and identify
the bodies from relatives who were to be flown into
Pristina the next day by WFP. I expressed grave
doubts about viewing bodies at this stage but UN
officials were pressing hard for this to be done if
the relatives insisted. Jo Greenfield [International
Nursing Advisor] arranged a viewing room with
appropriate décor and flowers. The UN were also
talking about a ceremony with the coffins altogether
and we arranged in the medical faculty for this
purpose. We were told that special air transport
coffins were en route.

The requirement for me to issue a certificate of
death and the obvious need to assess the suitability
of bodies for viewing and the likelihood of visual
identification meant that I should examine each of
the bodies.

The bodies arrived at the hospital, by
helicopter, at about 1600hrs. They were in body
bags. 24 bags contained remains clearly identifiable
as one victim. Bag 25 contained human remains that
had not yet been matched to a victim.

The bodies were naked. Given the known details of
the accident and my experience of these matters I
assumed their clothes had been removed at the scene.
(I was medical incident officer at Lockerbie where
bodies thrown from the aircraft at great height had
their clothes removed by the blast). The body bags
were numbered sequentially although with two
numbering systems. There was no accompanying

documentation. There were plastic bags containing some of the clothes that had obviously been cut off. Most of the bodies had no rings or jewellery.

I examined each of the bodies and Dr Hayden recorded my findings. It was clear that only two could reasonably be viewed and another two or three viewed after preparation by a skilled mortuary technician. We worked until late that night. In case of power cuts John Wood [International Director of Estates] arranged for emergency generators and lighting to the autopsy room.

Several UN officials attended that evening, each asking the same questions. I informed each visitor that the bodies would not be viewable and that identification would take some time. I told each UN official including Dr Chevalier, Dr Kouchner's assistant, that the bodies were naked and without personal effects or jewellery. No one knew this or could offer an explanation. I told each of them that the most likely explanation is that whoever was in charge of the scene arranged for this to be done and somewhere is all the personal effects and remaining clothes. In particular I told them that someone has all the documentation and ID cannot be completed until this is located and matched.

We resumed the work early the next day on Sunday 14/11/99. Two Gendarmes arrived at about 0900 and informed us they had been involved at the crash scene. They confirmed their clothes had been removed at the scene and that the numbers on the plastic bags of clothes did correspond to the numbers on the body bags. We could never establish why their clothes were removed at the scene. They brought with them all the personal jewellery and documentation which they had removed at the crash scene. Fortunately, this was in individual bags with numbers corresponding to the body bags and the clothing bags. At least 17 bodies could be identified fairly quickly by matching the documentation they had on their person.

During the morning I attended a meeting in Dr Kouchner's office. They had established a crisis group. At the meeting was Dr Kouchner, his assistant Dr Chevalier, Joc Covey Deputy SRSG, the Deputy Director of WFP, Maryon Bacharraut UN Director of Administration, Enrique Aguilar UN Regional Administrator for Pristina and a UN police officer. I informed them that the bodies would not be viewable and that ID would be completed by documentation. In spite of my repeated advice about the difficulties in viewing bodies it became clear that WFP had informed relatives that they would be able to see the bodies at the hospital. The Crisis group accepted my advice that viewing was to be avoided at this stage. I agreed to meet with the relatives at the airport on their arrival. Dr Kouchner was to address them and they would be flown over the crash site. Dr Kouchner informed the group that the Italian Government was pressing hard for the complete operation to be moved to Rome (12 of the victims were Italian). Forensic

autopsies on the crew and formal autopsies on the
passengers and all legal and identification
processes could be completed there. Dr Kouchner
clearly favoured this option. I advised that this
was a good option provided the process underway at
the hospital was completed and that all human
remains and documentation were moved together. Past
experience has shown serious problems can follow
when body parts and personal effects become
separated.

Meanwhile identification was progressing well by
documentation and Mr Aguilar and myself were
producing the medical certificates of death.[11]

On my way to the airport to meet with the
relatives we received a radio call from Dr Kouchner.
The bodies were to be taken to the airport at once
and be taken to Rome along with the relatives. I was
asked to turn back and supervise the operation. The
examination and documentation process were in fact
now complete but the coffins had only just arrived.
They were not special flight coffins. Nevertheless,
they were adequate for the short flight to Rome.

Two representatives from Kenyon's the
international funeral directors who specialise in
large disasters were now present. They had been
brought in by WFP to advise. Unfortunately, their
presence was never formally acknowledged by UNMIK
and they were unable to function in any official
capacity. This was a pity as they have all the
experience and contacts to facilitate the legal and

identification process including transport of
bodies. I know the organisation well and in fact I
knew the two representatives. They had worked with
me at Lockerbie. I emphasised their usefulness to
the crisis committee but to no real avail.

The bodies were taken to the airport arriving
after dark. The relatives' plane had already left.
The Italian air force pilot did not want to take off
in the dark and I understand the RAF ground staff
would not guarantee his safety if he did. I am told
he came under enormous pressure from the UN and that
eventually the Italian Ambassador from Belgrade
'persuaded' him to take off. The bodies were being
loaded on to the plane watched by colleagues of the
dead when everything stopped. It transpired that in
order to get the double body bags into the wooden
(non-flight) coffins, the US technicians had not
unreasonably removed the metal linings of the
coffins. The pilot was now insisting that these
linings be replaced and the metal edges be welded
together. He was saying that there is an
international law that requires coffins to be sealed
to prevent gases escaping and affecting the pressure
in the plane. The Kenyon's people knew nothing of
this regulation. I knew nothing of it. I cannot
understand how bodies so badly damaged could cause
any such threat. It was I believed a spurious excuse
to resist the pressure to fly. The coffins were
unloaded and we left. I heard later that Dr Kouchner
was summoned to the airport after midnight.

Colleagues of the dead were angry that the coffins were left standing on the ground of a tent and some better arrangements had to be made. The plane left the next day and no further problems have been reported to me.

I was asked to attend a press conference on Monday 15/11/99. This passed without incident from my point of view but the deputy director of WFP was subjected to very hostile questioning about the safety of the plane and the air traffic facilities at Pristina airport.

The memorial ceremony was held at the UNMIK building on Friday 19/11/99. Joc Covey gave an excellent homily and the ceremony was very well received. Official invitations were given to international and local hospital staff in recognition of their work and this was greatly appreciated.

The hospital I believe served three very useful functions.

It provided a base for the formal identification of the victims.

It provided the expertise for the initial examination of the victims.

It provided a focal point for activity.

There were difficulties and I've described them above. However, this is not to complain. I have dealt with many major incidents. It is in their nature that they are accompanied by confusion and high emotion and sometimes anger. The strength of

```
your response lies in how well you accommodate these
frustrations and difficulties. The UN community did
by and large come together and the efforts of the
hospital I believe were crucial to this. I have been
lobbying the UN for a formal major incident plan
prior to this event, which has now served to
concentrate minds on the urgency of this
requirement.
```

As my time in Kosovo came to a close, friends and colleagues began commenting on my continuing weight loss. Although I felt reasonably well, I was becoming fatigued again and the occasional muscle spasms that I had begun to experience, were to prove the herald of more ill health to come.

8.

Bringing the War Back Home

Gaza / Manchester / Sarajevo

Even if you never go to war, war can still come to you. It has come to us twice in Manchester in recent years. In 2017 in the rucksack of a suicide bomber at the Manchester Arena, and in 1996 courtesy of the IRA. When the latter happened, I was already in a war but home on leave. I was doing a clinic in the centre of Manchester with my colleague Dr Mark Prescott when we heard the noise of a helicopter overhead and a loudhailer telling us to vacate the area immediately. As we left the building, we heard the unmistakable sound of exploding ordnance, so familiar to me from Sarajevo, and saw the stream of debris hurtling sideways down the street that crossed in front of us. We grabbed our medical bags from our vehicles and ran towards the explosion where we set up and ran a First Aid post until the emergency services were on the scene.

War can come to you in less dramatic ways. It will creep into your home through your TV, lodge in your head through social media, and sometimes, whoever you may be, penetrate your heart. A senior civil servant told me that he was in 10 Downing Street briefing the then Prime Minister John Major, when they stopped to watch a TV news report from Bosnia on the plight of Irma

Hadzimuratovic, a five year-old girl severely injured by a mortar shell. Her Bosnian doctor, my erstwhile colleague in Sarajevo Dr Jganjac, was live on-air pleading for someone to offer her refuge and give her the treatment without which she would surely die. John Major muttered something to the effect of 'I wish there was something I could do,' to which the civil servant told me he replied, 'You *are* the Prime Minister, Sir.' He described how the PM's face lightened and said something like 'Indeed I am. Do whatever is necessary to bring her out of there and over here.' Forthwith, an RAF Hercules was promptly dispatched to airlift little Irma to London's Great Ormond Street Hospital. Although Irma improved, she never fully recovered, and sadly died eighteen months later, still in Great Ormond Street Hospital. Once again, questions were asked about was it all worth it for just one child? The same questions were raised about that little child rescued from the water, almost ten years previously. They always will be. Another 'gesture' perhaps, but not an altogether empty one.

It triggered a chain of events that led to many more children being evacuated from the horrors of Sarajevo than might otherwise have been the case had the world's attention, even for a moment, not been drawn through her to the plight of others. It also sent me back into Sarajevo for the third time that year. One week after Irma arrived on these shores, in August 1993, I was asked by the Emergency Aid Department of the ODA to deploy with my team to assist in the evacuation of further sick and injured patients. Despite what was written and said in the media at the time; there were no limits placed on the numbers we could rescue. Nor did we pick and choose at random those to be brought to safety in the UK. And neither did we leave anyone behind. John Major had been quite clear. 'Send a jumbo jet, if necessary,' I was told he said. I know for sure that additional planes were put on standby. When the war comes to you through the lens of a war photographer, or the microphone of a war reporter, your opinions are inevitably shaped by the views they and their editors have taken in shaping the piece you will see or read. There is always another view, and always a backstory.

A briefing from RAF Strike Command the following day suggested there would be no more than twenty patients destined for the UK, and each would be accompanied by at least two adults. En route to Stanstead airport the information about our patients changed continuously but I told the team not to worry and to be prepared for anything. When I was invited to join the United Nations Disaster Assessment and Coordination (UNDAC) team shortly after my work in Armenia, I naively asked about a job description. 'A high tolerance for ambiguity' was the only reply, and a more accurate job description than that I've never received – before or since. By their very nature, humanitarian emergencies are awash with uncertainties, and information, such as you can get, is often unreliable and forever changing. As important to any mission as the plans you make at the start is your ability to adapt them to the circumstances unfolding before you.

'Operation Irma', as our mission became known, attracted formidable press interest, which I described in my contemporaneous notes as 'frenetic'. But this was as nothing compared to what was yet to come. What seemed to me at the start as a straightforward humanitarian mission to evacuate children from a war-torn city under perpetual siege, turned rapidly into something very different. Two good doctors, each determined to do their best, had come head-to-head over the age-old medical conflict between doing the most for the most, and the most for the one in front of you. One, an RAF medical officer who had been into Sarajevo the day before to assess those already listed for evacuation by the UN, and the other a UN doctor based in Sarajevo and responsible for implementing the UN medical evacuation programme (MEDEVAC). The press reported the RAF doctor as saying he had major concerns about the composition of the evacuation list: about these being adults and not children, and adults who seemed to him to be wounded soldiers. This now threw petrol onto the bonfire of the media. We had in fact asked that a wider team be deployed on that first RAF foray into Sarajevo, in order to include those who had previous experience of working in their hospitals. But the British military did not agree. However, given what had unfolded, at a subsequent meeting it was agreed that myself, a senior paediatrician in our team, and the RAF medical officer (also a paediatrician) would go back into Sarajevo, and this time be accompanied by a Ministry of Defence press officer and our translator (the one from my very first mission to Sarajevo the year before). We would review the list of evacuees and arrange for their transfer to the airport and onwards to the UK. A final phone call to the UN doctor in Sarajevo indicated that there would now be a further four children for evacuation, including a child with paralysis of both legs, and Belma, a young girl with meningitis.

The medical evacuation of children from a war zone seems an obviously good thing to do, but it can be fraught with difficulties. Emotions run high across the press and public, and at times it has seemed to me, with little tolerance or understanding of the obstacles to overcome. Children will need to be accompanied, ideally by their parents. But how can you separate them from their siblings? So, it is never just one child. It is several people, including adults. But governments in war zones may not want their adult citizens, particularly men of fighting age, to leave. If ethnic cleansing is in the conflict mix, as it was in Sarajevo, then medical evacuation may be seen by their government as to serendipitously contribute. Accepting a child for treatment is often, therefore, just the start of what can be a long and byzantine bureaucratic process with their own government to secure their permission to leave. And what if their parents are dead? Who then gives permission, and who else should accompany the child? What if the parents are assumed to be dead, but are in fact still alive, somewhere else?

Over ten years later, while working in the aftermath of the earthquake in Haiti, my team was asked to review a child in a local field hospital. This tiny infant we were told was orphaned in the earthquake and had been found by rescuers in the ruins of a hospital. She had incurred terrible injuries, including the loss of an arm, and wounds to the head and scalp. We had a plastic surgeon in our team who was asked to surgically explore the wound to the scalp, clean out the infection, and repair it as much as possible. With the operation successfully completed she was safely returned to the referring field hospital. I next heard of the baby one month later. I read she had been evacuated by a charity to a hospital in London, and was now having further treatment to her scalp injury there. But once in the UK it emerged gradually that she was neither orphaned by, nor injured in, the earthquake. Her mother was found to be alive, living in Haiti, and grieving for the missing child she presumed to be dead. She was able to explain that her baby was already in the hospital before the earthquake, following a fall into the fire at home. She had burned her arm so badly that it needed amputating; the wounds to her scalp were poorly treated burns. When she went to the hospital after the earthquake, she'd found it to be in ruins and her child to be missing, presumed dead. Despite the very best of intentions, many stones need to be turned before a child can be safely assumed to be an orphan in the chaos of a major disaster. Happily in this case mother and child were reunited..

And when the treatment is complete, what then? Can, or even should, they be returned to the area of conflict? If children stay until the war is over, this can often mean them doing their growing up in another country, speaking another language, and integrating into another culture. Going back from whence they came may no longer be going home but leaving.

Medical evacuation to the UK is not always the best solution if somewhere nearer, and importantly culturally similar, is willing to help. In 2014 the team was asked by the British Government to fly into Gaza and assess what help may be required in the aftermath of the recent conflict, and if there were patients who might benefit from transfer to the UK for further treatment. What they found was that, as is so often the case, the local staff had dealt with the immediate life-threatening injuries, but outside support was required for their longer-term rehabilitation. With our partner NGO Humanity and Inclusion, we ran a six months rehabilitation programme for the war injured in Gaza. Importantly, we could feed back to the authorities in the UK that patients who might benefit from treatment elsewhere had already been evacuated locally, and to Arabic speaking countries. Putting aid into a country to support a patient's treatment there rather than taking them out may be preferable to some, but not all. There are many who quite reasonably, simply want out. Not everyone will be allowed out by their country or accepted by another, and the human trading that follows can be a dreadful and distressing experience for all concerned.

On arrival in Sarajevo I spoke with UN officials who I noted in my diary to be 'clearly upset and distressed about the apparent conflict that had developed between the UN (in Sarajevo) and the British government' over who should be evacuated. Of course this was more a conflict between two people rather than between an international organisation and a country. Whilst the RAF doctor was complaining to the press about the composition of the evacuation list, the UN doctor was quoted in *The Times* of London as saying Britain was launching a 'public relations exercise' and treating children like 'zoo animals'. And there was I in the middle. *The Times* went further, and quoted an unknown 'senior British official,' said to have 'been involved in the evacuation,' as saying there was 'no doubt that money is changing hands to get soldiers out, while children are being left behind.' There are two elements to this. I have no proof, but would not be surprised if money was changing hands at some point in the chain. People were desperate, and those with influence were certainly using their power and position to jump the queue. The little girl whose plight had triggered the situation we now all found ourselves in may have earned her place on the RAF Hercules one week earlier as much by her being a close relative of a member of the Bosnian government as by the desperate state of her health. She needed and benefited from the help that was given to her, but I am equally alive to the brutalities of war, and what people will do to save their own – especially the lives of their loved ones. Moreover the political connections that thrust her into the spotlight allowed this light to spread into a corner of the war where nobody wanted to look. The desperate plight of the children in Sarajevo was painful to see, but we must never look away. The other element – the evacuation of soldiers over children – we addressed face-on with the UN and Bosnian authorities. It is also easy to make assumptions based on appearances alone. This unknown source quoted in the paper went on later to describe several of the potential evacuees as wearing military trousers or shirts, and 'suffering from typical combat wounds that would be obvious to the doctors who examined them in Britain.' I never found out who the person was, but anyone with experience of working in Sarajevo would have been familiar with the wounding of civilians with combat weapons. Wearing camouflage shirts and trousers in a hospital in an active war zone is fairly common. They may of course have been soldiers, but they may also have been civilians dressed in the only clothing available to them after their bloodied and torn garments had been removed by their treating doctors. In an emergency department in the UK, having cut off all the clothes of a motorcyclist without moving him to examine for hidden injuries, I sent him home later dressed in surgical scrubs, with his clothes cut to ribbons in a plastic bag. This did not make him a surgeon. These observations, made without qualification, proved little either way to the knowledgeable. But they added yet more fuel to what was now a blazing fire.

Once in Sarajevo, I began exploring with all those involved, how the humanitarian mission to evacuate children that I thought I'd embarked upon had now suddenly morphed into an airlift of combatants. On the one side was the UN medical evacuation, MEDEVAC, committee that applied a set of principles, agreed with the Bosnian government, to identify the most urgent and suitable cases. On the other side was an individual who had found mainly adults on the evacuation list, and having toured the wards, declared there were still children there who were suitable for evacuation to the UK. Whilst acting in an essentially individual capacity, these actions were interpreted as being those of the British government, which was now accused of 'cherry picking'. The UN MEDEVAC protocol was in fact open to all ages, and the UN was at pains to point out that the Geneva Conventions required all combatants to be viewed as civilians once they had been wounded. To be clear, international humanitarian law draws no distinction between civilians and combatants once they are wounded and withdrawn from the field of battle ('hors de combat'). Whether you like it or not, if there were wounded soldiers on the evacuation list, they had the same right in law to be there as the sick and injured children as long as it could be justified by the severity and urgency of their medical condition. I couldn't see the argument garnering much sympathy from a press and public now on a mission to save the wounded children of Sarajevo.

The crisis reached its peak when the RAF declared there would be no evacuation at all if there were any Bosnian military personnel on the plane. This would make the plane a legitimate military target and the Serbs would shoot it down. I had in fact had similar arguments put to me by the RAF before we left Ancona in Italy to fly into Sarajevo. Again, there are two elements to this concern. Would their presence make the plane a target and would it be a legitimate target? To the occupants of the aircraft, whether the Serbs considered it a legitimate target was of little concern. I had been on the airlift many times when chaff was discharged from the aircraft as it took off to divert incoming missiles, so I knew he had a point. It was already a target. Given the disregard for international humanitarian law occurring daily by the shelling and shooting of civilians, if they knew there were Bosnian soldiers on board, I expect it could have made it even more of a target. But it wasn't a legitimate target and I believed what he was saying to be wrong. He went further, though, and said that he would cancel the evacuation now if the list of evacuees remained unchanged. This was perceived as against international humanitarian law and now too much for the UN doctor who picked up the phone to make a pre-emptive strike and cancel the mission himself. We onlookers somehow managed to persuade them both to take a step back and agree to take me and my colleagues to see for ourselves the patients put up for evacuation. On arrival at the hospital the media were lying in wait for us and barking questions that we felt we couldn't, perhaps shouldn't, answer until we had seen all the patients. Here was a perfect storm of seemingly irreconcilable viewpoints, emanating from those in high office in the UN and British Military, but to be played out on the frontline of the Bosnian war. Witness to it all, and with their own views, were the media, who while like us were risking their lives to be in Sarajevo, were there to tell a story and get a picture. If they couldn't, I often sensed they felt that risking their life here was ultimately futile. And in this tinderbox dry environment, if we didn't let them accompany us around the hospital, or listen to our private conversations with patients, they thought we surely must have something to hide.

Being under fire in Sarajevo was bad enough but being attacked by the media made it unbearable for some. The UN doctor was particularly distressed about the reports in the press implying that he personally was refusing or delaying the evacuation of patients, without recognising his entrapment between the twin bureaucracies of the UN and the local Bosnian authorities. I took him to one side and tried my best to reassure him that I for one knew he was acting in good faith and would always ensure I told his side of the story. He broke down and wept uncontrollably. The unbearable strain of the last few weeks and months; the constant risk to his own life from shells and snipers; the pouring through lists of desperate souls; the invidious choices; the personal threats from patients' relatives; and now the fear of now being judged by the world as more Mengele than Schweitzer – all these came tumbling out in a flood of utter helplessness.[12]

We toured the University Hospital and agreed all those in need of immediate evacuation were in fact already on the list. Tensions around if any of these were possible (ex-)combatants eased in the decompression chamber of dialogue. On leaving, we were once again ambushed in a circle of cameras and reporters. Although we had agreed as a group with the Ministry of Defence press officer to say nothing to the press as we left, like a pride of hunting lions they picked off the RAF officer, weakened they sensed by him already having spoken to them, and having separated him from the group, secured another interview. The rest of us went on to the other hospital in Sarajevo, the infamous 'Swiss Cheese' hospital, so called because of its multiple shell holes, and previously a military hospital. While the Ministry of Defence press officer stood guard at the entrance to ward off any advancing predators, we entered the hospital and met with Dr Jganjac.

In this work you quickly learn that things are never exactly as they seem. Dr Jganjac had gained his place on the television news as much through his connections with the Bosnian government as through his role as a surgeon. Those who stayed in Sarajevo, either by choice or usually by force, suffered terribly. I saw it in Dr Jganjac. He had lost so much weight in the few months since I saw him last. I noted too how he was breathless when climbing the stairs in hospital – so different to the robust young man that drove me speeding in his car down Sniper Alley six months earlier. Rekindling our friendship, he confided in me that the UN had refused to listen to his pleas to evacuate Irma. Although there was a MEDEVAC committee, it met infrequently he complained, as its members were often all away at the same time. He had become frustrated by their lack of the ability to make decisions in an emergency, and asked me to understand that was why he'd gone to the media. Of course in so doing he had undermined the UN and its attempts to make MEDEVAC an objective process, free from influence. He repeated some of these concerns in open discussion, but the UN countered quickly with reference to the clumsy bureaucracy of the local government, with which of course he was closely associated. Amid the traded blows, I discovered a simple but major hurdle to what at times appeared to be a Kafkaesque procedure. Photographs of each applicant were required by the Bosnian government to accompany each application. But this was pre-mobile phones, when cameras were not in everybody's pocket. Even digital cameras were yet to replace film in Sarajevo at that time. I made a note to self to supply both the UN and the Bosnian government with Polaroid cameras. In the end we had a long, frank and fruitful discussion with Dr Jganjac and the UN doctor, and our presence appeared to facilitate a much calmer discussion. My notes at the time record that I was convinced they'd left with a better understanding of each other's unenviable position. We learned that eighty-seven patients had been evacuated in the previous few months since the UN MEDEVAC committee had become operational. There were still 435 cases waiting to be processed, sixty-five of whom had eye problems. I made a note of this too and included the provision of eye surgery in a later aid programme that I ran in Sarajevo.

Back at the University Hospital we were reunited with the RAF officer. He was very concerned for the welfare of Belma, the little girl with meningitis, who I learned he had successfully added to the list on his first visit, the day before. We considered organising her immediate evacuation but given the even worse insecurity of Sarajevo at night, this was abandoned as being simply not feasible.

Rather than travel through the blacked-out sniper ridden city, we prepared to spend the night in the UN office within the University Hospital grounds. Trying to settle down to get some sleep on the floor of the office, on a stiflingly hot Sarajevo summer evening, we were startled by a sudden noise of movement outside. We kept very still and silent and were beginning to be afraid until we heard the sing-song chanting of English voices outside shouting 'we know you're in there, we know you're in there.' The relief that it wasn't armed soldiers was instant, followed almost as quickly by a feeling of unreality at the incongruity of the playground scenario we could hear but not yet see. Tentatively opening the door, we discovered that it was a British television camera crew who, unbeknown to us, had been told by the RAF Officer to meet us there at 9pm. We managed, I think, to explain to them the importance and sensitivity of our mission and how patients' needs and privacy dictated our approach to the media. Feeling somewhat vulnerable now though, we managed to secure an escort to the UN PTT building, where once again we tried to get some sleep on the floor.

These evacuations from war zones are never simple, and those who shout that 'something must be done' must realise also that in so doing, they may also be shouting 'and someone may likely die'. The transfer of patients within Sarajevo and on to the dangerous area of the airport was organised and run admirably by the French military. I was to learn later that a local UN worker assisting with the exercise was shot dead by a sniper. We ourselves came under fire from snipers as we boarded the plane with our patients.

The journey home was to be in two stages. The first by RAF Hercules from Sarajevo into the Italian coastal town of Ancona, where we had positioned a team in a temporary hospital, and then by an ODA chartered aircraft to the UK. As we had feared, on leaving Sarajevo, Belma was very ill and required continuous intensive care during the transfer to the UK. Our anaesthetist, Dr Peter Oakley, did a most remarkable job, and kept her sedated and on a ventilator for the whole of the journey. She arrived at her final destination stable and in a better condition than we had found her in Sarajevo. Our first stop was London, where we were met by a procession of ambulances and from where Belma went to join Irma in Great Ormond Street Hospital. We had deliberately sized our team to enable us to peel off team members for each of the patients we distributed and to continue their care in transit to the receiving hospital. We travelled on to Birmingham and then to Leeds to distribute the remaining patients. As the plane bunny-hopped between cities in the UK, I smiled at the children, pulling funny faces and playing hide and seek between the seats. I looked too at the contrasting weary faces of their parents, each showing a complex mixture of emotions. They portrayed relief at knowing they were now out of the horror Sarajevo and their children would get the treatment they so desperately needed; anxiety for the unknown that lay ahead for them in a country they did not know; and a fear and sadness for all those, and all that, they had left behind. It is never easy to leave everything you have ever known, even your language, behind in a country being destroyed by war. Many do, and usually for the sake of their children, but do not underestimate the bravery it requires.

With all the patients safely delivered to their respective hospitals I made my way back to my NHS hospital to resume my NHS clinical work.

Why use a civilian aircraft once back in the UK, you might ask? The correspondence I saw later revealed that the RAF were to charge the ODA for its most suitable aircraft, a VC10, £3475 per hour. For the 72 hours of the mission this would have amounted to £271,000 (over half a million pounds in today's money). This was 3.5 times the £76,000 the ODA had negotiated to hire a Russian Tupolev and an unnecessary, and unjustifiable, bite out of the limited aid budget for the mission. This is in general why aid agencies, including DFID, choose civilian over military resources. Government departments are required to charge each other for the use of services, even when the money is ultimately all coming out of the same taxpayer's pot. Whilst this might appear to be a paper exercise, it is so much more. Moving the money from one budget to another is of course reducing the size of the donor's budget which has a much wider knock-on effect, particularly in overseas aid. When the government agrees to support a humanitarian programme, a fixed amount of money is agreed. From that everything required to deliver the aid is drawn. It is morally incumbent upon us all to ensure that as much of that money is spent on the humanitarian needs of the affected population. As much as some politicians would like, it is not for me to see it being spent back here in the UK any more than is absolutely necessary, under the pretence of overseas aid supporting domestic programmes that should have been appropriately funded in the first place.

There was to be one last sting for me in the tail of 'Operation Irma'. A newspaper had run pictures of a young girl they claimed had been left behind by my team in Sarajevo, 'screaming in pain from a brain tumour.' The child had no such thing; she had a severe and long-standing disability, was well cared for in the hospital, and neither the staff, and most importantly nor her parents, had asked for her to be evacuated. The story I learned had been given to a journalist by someone in the hospital, either ignorant of the diagnosis or looking to keep the pressure on for more evacuations. But the story was damaging. I was asked by a government official to speak with a rival newspaper that was willing to run with my rebuttal, to which I somewhat foolishly agreed. I pulled back though after some reflection, and after colleagues in the team had reminded me that I was at risk of breaking medical confidences. I then received a phone call at work from the newspaper. They were less than pleased, had prepared their story, and were not willing to see a chance to get one over on a newspaper rival get away without a fight. I tried my best to explain my position, somewhat weakened by having originally agreed, when he said, 'we can make life very difficult for you, you know?'

I did know. I was terrified. It is every doctor's nightmare to be doorstepped by journalists, to have their professional and private lives raked over without mercy. A doctor's most precious possession is their reputation. It is so hard fought for and so easily lost. Nevertheless, I had to try now and be the good doctor, place my patient's interests above mine, and stick to my guns. I put down the phone and imagined my life and career about to be torn to shreds. But nothing happened. It took a few fearful days and sleepless nights for me to be sure, but the storm seemed to have passed. I did write letters of riposte to editors, but held back on any details, and lived to fight another day.

That day came quite quickly. On Friday 17 December 1993 I received another call from the ODA asking the team to support the UN International Organisation for Migration (IOM) in the evacuation to the UK of children from Mostar. 'Operation Angel', was so called because of the involvement of the 'Angel of Mostar' Sally Becker. But without the direct involvement of the British government, and the inevitable, and often potentially hostile, press pack that follows, this passed relatively quietly, and certainly without the furore that had surrounded 'Operation Irma'.

*

If you do go to war, you will always bring a bit of the war back home with you. This will be in memories, usually bad, but sometimes good, and in the nightmares that can follow. Whenever I was home from humanitarian missions to Sarajevo, I was haunted by what I'd seen; and any rest ruined by my dread of having to go back. I say having to go. I was always an unpaid volunteer, but I had made a commitment: to people in that beleaguered city; to colleagues who'd stepped forwards with me to help; and to myself. I had to see it through. Most of the time I could cope, and each time I settled temporarily back into life in the UK, my tension eased.

But I wasn't prepared for Bonfire Nights. These became unbearable. On the first 5 November back in the UK, I was driving home from my clinical work at the hospital when the fireworks began to go off. I immediately and spontaneously went onto high alert. I tried to tell myself these noises were not snipers and shells, but people simply enjoying themselves. But my anxiety grew more and more, until I became extremely angry. I swore loudly into the empty car, banging the steering wheel with my fist, and screaming into the night that such things are not toys. How could people be so stupid? I had to pull the car over into a layby. The noises and the flashes wouldn't go away; I could feel myself gasping for air and my heart bursting in my chest. I slowly pulled myself together as best I could. Tears were now rolling down my red-hot cheeks as I leaned over the steering wheel and tried to reassure myself. To tell myself everything is okay. And then another, even more powerful fear emerged. I must not, could not, allow myself to think these things;

that such sights and sounds were only toys and fireworks. I was going back to where they were very much for real. So, I swallowed the tension and kept it there, deep inside, year upon year. I had to assume that any sudden crack was the shot of a sniper; that I mustn't walk near open windows to avoid snipers and bomb blast; that I must avoid the grass verges by the roadside, for that is where they bury antipersonnel mines. I had to stay scared to stay safe. My family learned quickly that bonfire night, or indeed any other fireworks celebration, was not for me. I stayed inside the house under the pretence of looking after the cat, while they each took turns to pretend that they'd had enough of the fireworks and fancied coming inside for a while to sit quietly by my side.

Travelling regularly in and out of Sarajevo for almost four years, particularly on the airlift, was a source of great anxiety for me, no doubt enhanced by the shooting down of the Italian aircraft only a few weeks after I had first flown on it. But surprisingly, once in Sarajevo, I could at times experience a peculiar calm. Life was terrifying, brutal, and hard. But there was a hyperreality – a heightened sense of awareness, kindled by knowing that any day you might die, but this day you didn't. Not all the time, but enough to almost make being there a dangerous source of refuge. Life there was simpler. You lived in the most basic of accommodation, eating the rations you brought in with you, and each day usually only going to and from the hospital. The strains of everyday living, looking after children, paying the household bills, all that remained at home to be managed by others. And those of us in the city, like many who find themselves in similar situations, tried to force a normality on the abnormal life we were leading. One morning in the emergency department after a night of particularly heavy shelling, I met a group of Bosnian medical students who had fought their way to the hospital at great risk to their lives to attend their scheduled teaching. I explained to them that the hospital was now extremely busy and I'd been told to tell them that no one would be available to teach them. Their faces lit up. To shouts of 'dobro!' they were gone.

We did try to have some downtime, but this was always ruined by the intrusion of war. One of the anaesthetists who I became friends with told me he played classical guitar. I played blues guitar and he said he'd always wanted to learn. So, we agreed to try and teach other the basics of the two techniques. He invited me to his apartment after work on a lovely summer's late afternoon. I remember him opening the French windows and inviting me to join him on the balcony to play the guitar and enjoy the evening sunshine. His wife became extremely anxious. She said very nervously that he knew there was a sniper in the nearby hillside who targeted these apartments and we should stay inside. He seemed embarrassed at her countering his invitation and said there had been no shooting for at least a few days, moved two chairs onto the balcony, and invited me to join him. I have always been disappointed by how easily my natural tendency to self-survival and mantra of stay scared, stay safe, can be immediately suppressed by my greater fear of social embarrassment. So, I joined him. His wife stayed inside. At first it seemed as though her anxieties may have been misplaced, until a series of small columns of dust ran across the balcony edge in front of us, left to right, as machine-gun fire raked across a metre or so in front of us. His wife screamed in terror and we dived back together through the French windows and onto the floor. A few more sporadic shots rang out and then no more. We were shaking and his wife was in tears. Angry with our neglect and angry with herself for not stopping us. The sniper could have killed us and was showing us that he could. Such is terror. If you kill everyone who ventures out then no one ventures out. But kill enough to keep fear and terror in the population, but not enough to stop everything moving, then each day you face the agony of deciding if it's worth it, and the guilt of living with the consequences when you find out that it wasn't.

The souvenirs of war are physical, tangible, as well as psychological. The maimed and missing limbs; the scars and disability. Most of these are manifest from the time they leave the field of battle. I never got a war wound as such. The nearest I came to one was when I was asleep on a sofa and a mortar exploded just outside. The shock and the noise caused me to sit bolt upright, still half asleep. I quickly checked myself over and realised I was okay, but before I could settle back, a large painting that had been hanging on the wall, had unknown to me in the dark of a Sarajevo blackout, become dislodged by the blast and was teetering on its hook. As I realised how lucky I was to be alive and uninjured, it fell silently, and hit me on the head. Even then I was lucky. I wasn't hit by the heavy frame; but rather by the rough surface of the canvas as it scraped down the side of my face. I had quite an impressive abrasion, which however proved to be very superficial, and almost to my disappointment, healed without scarring.

*

For me the wounds of war were to grow quietly, gradually; but terribly. By the time I was finishing my later work in Kosovo I was already experiencing cramps in my abdomen, not just inside but also clearly in the muscle. While these gradually grew worse, I was able to continue with consultancy work. I even had one or two more humanitarian missions, including Sierra Leone during the civil war as part of the United Nations Disaster Assessment and

Coordination Team, and the following year a mission to Kenya in the aftermath of the Nairobi bombing. But by then I realised all was not well. I was losing weight again. I had also begun to experience progressive, severe widespread stiffness, and worryingly, several other neurological symptoms. The abdominal tightness progressed into obvious jerks and then came the spasms of the arms and legs. I was extremely self-conscious of these spontaneous jerks and found their psychological impact on me extremely distressing – worse even than their associated physical discomfort. By the time I saw a neurologist I was walking very stiffly and with difficulty and had almost continuous rhythmic spasms of the abdominal muscles (myoclonus). I had also developed a highly abnormal startle response, which I still have to some degree to this day. Any sudden noise would cause me to go suddenly and perfectly rigid, my arms and legs extended in a bizarre star jump. Once when I was at home, while at the top of the stairs, I felt myself lose my balance and my sudden movement towards the handrail triggered a marked startle response so severe that it caused me to completely flatten out. I slid down the stairs like a tin tray, landing at the bottom shocked, but remarkably uninjured.

When I saw a neurologist, he was confident that I had Moersch Woltman syndrome, also known as stiff person syndrome, a rare neurological disorder with an underlying autoimmune basis. However, there was one other important diagnosis to rule out: motor neurone disease. This would be diagnosed by an electrical test of the muscles.

The neurologist who did the test was kind and sensitive to my medical knowledge and corresponding anxiety. He went straight to the relevant part of the test and before he'd completed all that he had to do, looked up and said it's not motor neurone disease. I need to do a few more things to find out what it is, but I wanted you to know. As much as I was relieved, I couldn't help also thinking about all those others who had lay on that same couch and been told something very different. As my illness deteriorated and people would say how unlucky I was, I always found myself saying 'You're wrong, I'm very lucky that it wasn't something else.'

I discussed the fear I felt of it being motor neurone disease with my neurologist. He understood, he said: 'There were worse diseases even than cancer.' At first perhaps an odd thing to say, but it made sense to me. We automatically think of cancer as the worst thing that can happen to us, and view those who work in the specialty as having one of the most difficult of jobs. In many ways, of course, this is correct. But cancer is now more a disease of later years, with obvious exceptions. Treatments are improving and it is no longer an automatic death sentence. As a neurologist, however, he had to tell people, often young people, of things that had no cure, and a death that would be as inevitable as it would be lingering. If the way he looked after me is anything to go by, then as difficult as their burden would be to carry, I knew they would be in the hands of someone who would do all they could to lighten the load.

Blood tests further confirmed the diagnosis of stiff person syndrome. I also now had signs and symptoms of a wider autoimmune disease affecting the kidney and my immune system. I knew from my work in the Balkans that there was a condition known as Balkans nephropathy. This had been thought at one time to be due to heavy metal poisoning, which was a recognised problem in the Balkans, where lead contaminated the water supply. While I was in Kosovo, Roma children in the north of the province had died of lead poisoning. It continues to be a health risk today. I also knew that my cluster of symptoms, particularly abdominal pain and neurological abnormalities, were suggestive of lead poisoning. I shared my concerns with my consultants, who carried out blood and urine tests but found no trace of lead or other heavy metals. When my health deteriorated quite significantly, I was admitted to hospital for immunoglobulin therapy. Liver and kidney biopsies were also performed and showed substantial deposits of lead and uranium, as well as other heavy metals including mercury. So, there it was: heavy metal poisoning. I certainly had an underlying chronic autoimmune disease, but it had been significantly exacerbated by poisoning. The poisoning, though, was not very recent, otherwise it would have been associated with detectable levels of lead in the blood and/or urine. Instead the heavy metals were lodged in high quantities in my liver and kidney. In the liver as they were ingested, and in the kidney as they were excreted. Just as 'adjuvants' are added to vaccines to stimulate the immune reaction, so the heavy metals now in my body stimulated an already vulnerable immune system and precipitated a widespread autoimmune disease that included the stiff person syndrome. To get the heavy metals out I embarked upon a programme of chelation therapy. This involved being admitted to hospital for one week a month over several months, where I was attached to a drip and given the chemical calcium sodium edetate. This had quite an impact on my daily life, but it was worth it, as the tests showed the stiff person syndrome antibody levels coming down as the metals were excreted. Gradually my symptoms were improving.

However, the chemical that removed the heavy metals could not distinguish between those metals we wanted out and those, particularly calcium, that we wanted to remain. Unfortunately, as my calcium levels fell so my bones became thin. So there came a point when I had to completely stop taking the chelation therapy and live with these Balkan souvenirs lodged deep in my internal organs.

There had been widespread concern about the use of depleted uranium in NATO weapons during the Balkans conflict. However, those who analysed my tissue samples concluded that they were consistent not with depleted uranium from ordnance, but with enriched, fissile uranium. So how did it happen? Well nobody knows for sure. I may have been first exposed to lead poisoning while working in Sarajevo, but I expect my illness then was my underlying autoimmune disease. However, lead poisoning in Kosovo is well established, and there is no doubt I became much more ill during my time there, and very ill on leaving. Certainly, during my early days there, the food that I could get was of dubious origin and could well have been grown in areas contaminated by the illegal disposal of nuclear waste in that unregulated land. This could have accounted for the ingestion of enriched uranium. But there is another possibility, and one that I have tried not to think about. Why was it only me, and why the combination of metals? Is it possible that I was poisoned deliberately? There were those who wanted to see me leave, and poisoning is not an unknown method of dealing with perceived troublemakers, particularly in that part of the world. Deliberate poisoning has been suggested to me on several occasions, and each time I have sought to reject it. There is no absolute proof and it could have been accidental. But I am increasingly persuaded, and recall being acutely ill while in Kosovo. I realise, too, that my reluctance to entertain it before was perhaps because I find it too hard to think that somebody could bear me such ill will. This came to the surface when I was interviewed by the BBC for a health programme that was exploring the targeting of humanitarian workers. During my pre-broadcast discussion with the researcher, I mentioned the heavy metal poisoning, and in response to a direct question, I intimated that there was a possibility that this may have been deliberate. When I was interviewed by the presenter the following day and this was again put to me, I was surprised how I just froze. I mumbled something and moved away from the topic. I emailed the researcher immediately afterwards and asked if she would explain to the presenter that until then I had never publicly faced up to the possibility of someone wishing to do me so much harm, and the reality of it had stopped me in my tracks. Not long afterwards I received a nice email from the presenter, Claudia Hammond, who reassured me, said she understood, and wished me well. It was an unexpected and very kind thing to do.

Whether deliberately or accidentally, there is no doubt that I was poisoned. Once confirmed I contacted the Department for International Development in case others in the team had been affected (I was the only case) and for them to raise awareness of it with the World Health Organisation. I was referred to their outsourced occupational health department who did little more than interview me over the phone. I spoke with colleagues at WHO, who said they were aware of heavy metal poisoning in the region, but said that this was mainly confined to children, and in particular children in the Roma community. In one piece of correspondence from a senior person in DFID there was even the suggestion that the Roma habit of giving lead diluted in water to cure sickness might be a factor in the local community.

But none of this explained how I became contaminated. I tried hard to get an investigation going, wider than the public health approach that was being adopted in Kosovo, and to secure funds for this from DFID, but to no avail. I put together an international team of kidney experts, and as suggested by DFID, I spoke with

WHO and with Dr Pleurat Sejdiu, who I knew well from my time in Kosovo, and who was still their Minister of Health. Both agreed that the methods they currently had in place did not detect the true prevalence of heavy metal poisoning in the Balkans and that there was an urgent need for further investigation, and the study I was planning was urgently required. DFID wrote to me saying that WHO now planned to propose a regional study and that it would be appropriate for them to make a 'modest contribution'. The letter concluded 'I hope that it will be able to provide us with greater understanding of this issue'. One year later I received a further letter from them saying that the Ministry of Health in Kosovo did not consider further work on this to be a high priority for additional funding:

> Within the region WHO considers that there is no compelling case for funding for the work and heavy metal poisoning; it is not a priority health need for the majority of people, nor specifically for the health needs of the poor … DFID allocates funds with the aim of ensuring the greatest possible impact in reducing poverty … While increased knowledge of the relative merits of kidney biopsy and blood tests as well as possible improvement of diagnostic techniques are laudable goals, they are not currently major public health priorities in the region. As a result, we are unable to support further scientific study.

Shortly after I received the letter, and unprompted, I received a call from a colleague in WHO with whom I was working on the study. She was worried there may have been some confusion in a call they'd had the week before with DFID, she said and wanted to reassure me that while WHO did not wish to carry out the research themselves, they fully supported the project I was proposing. I wrote again to DFID saying: 'I hope there's simply been some confusion and that DFID is not reneging on a commitment made against a background of what for me has been the devastating consequences of working for them in the Balkans.' There was no response.

After the immunotherapy and chelation therapy my health was much improved. I was back working full-time. We even published details of my case in *The Lancet*. The title we gave the paper was 'autoimmune diathesis precipitated by exposure to heavy metals.' It was published as 'A man who brought the war home with him.'

The stiffness continued and there were residual intermittent jerks, but I'd lost any embarrassment about them and people either didn't notice or were simply too kind to say. But the illness had a long tail, as I was to discover. The disease itself had left me more vulnerable to infections and its treatment left me more vulnerable to fractures. The price I was to pay for the work that I have done was set to rise even higher.

9.
Reading My Own Obituary

Cape Verde / China / Kenya / Mongolia / Sarajevo / Sierra Leone

It's a common fantasy, I believe, to wish to read your own obituary. In 2001 I almost did. As part of my commitment to the United Nations Disaster Assessment and Co-ordination (UNDAC) Team, I had been asked to go to Mongolia for a month to report on the impact of a steadily unfolding climate-related disaster. Working for UNDAC is unpaid and its team members are volunteers. Member countries nominate experts from a variety of backgrounds, and if they are accepted, they commit to paying for their training and deployment. I would have gone to Mongolia. A colleague had been there previously and spoke movingly of its people and their needs. However, when they moved the date of the mission, I found I was already committed to working in Kenya for an NGO and that this would now begin before the month's work required for the Mongolian mission would be completed. I had to decline, and my place was taken by another British member of the UNDAC Team.

Before I left for Kenya, I took a call from a colleague in the UN. I knew this would be no ordinary call when he asked me where I was, if I had anybody with me and if I would like to sit down. I sensed that whatever he was about to tell me was not going to be good, but I did not know just how bad it would be. Gerard Le Claire, the young family man who had taken my place on the mission, was dead. He was killed when the UN helicopter in which he was travelling crashed in the frozen wastes of Mongolia. Alongside him died my friend and colleague, Sabine Metzner-Strack, the team leader. Sabine and I were founder members of UNDAC and trained together in Geneva in 1993, in between my missions to Sarajevo. She had a young family at that time and told me she would be delaying her deployment overseas until they were older. Six others died alongside them, including another two UN workers.

I put the phone down and stared into space. That could have – should have – been me. More than relief, I felt guilt. A profound guilt for not going, and shame for allowing someone else to die in my place. I turned on the television and the radio, waiting for the news of these tragic deaths, to hear what they said about a young British man who had lost his life while engaged in voluntary humanitarian work for his country. But it never made it to the TV news. I never saw it in the newspapers. It figured only briefly, for no more than a few hours it seemed, on the internet and Ceefax, the BBC's then teletext service. Of far more concern to the BBC was the news that the Queen Mother had stumbled (not fallen) and received no injury. This was the top news story on the TV and radio in the UK for the twenty-four hours it took to retrieve Gerard's body from the snow and inform his young wife and children of his – and now their – sacrifice.

Since 2016, each year in August on World Humanitarian Day, there is a memorial service held at Westminster Abbey to remember and honour those humanitarian workers who have lost their lives while helping others. Afterwards we are invited to place a white rose on the ground and say out loud the names of those we wish to remember. As I place my flowers, I release the names of Gerard and Sabine into the London evening air. Their lives and sacrifice will never be forgotten, and certainly not by me.

I had in fact already experienced an earlier brush with my own obituary. In Sarajevo, a journalist rang me asking for details of where I was born, what school I went to, and other aspects of my life. Eventually it dawned on me just what they were doing. I stopped the conversation and said to the journalist 'are you writing my obituary?' There followed a silence that lasted just a little too long, then came words to the effect of, 'well it's always good to have these things on record.' I tried to make light of it and said something in response like 'well then, let's make sure it's accurate', but it was a brutal reminder to me of the risks I was taking. I had a very young family at the time, and I was already riddled with doubts about whether I had the right to risk their future by risking my own. I know there are those who would have made a different choice, and I know those who did choose differently. I know too there are those who consider the choice I made then to be wrong. Selfish even. Certainly reckless. But for good or for bad, I carried on.

When Sabine and I joined the United Nations Disaster Assessment and Coordination Team, (UNDAC), we were signing up to something new, something that was looking to improve the response to humanitarian crises. There is much goodwill ignited by a sudden catastrophic event. Much more than is generated by the chronic lingering humanitarian crises to which we can all become numbed, depressingly quickly. But at least it is doing something for someone. I've always worked on the basis that just because I can't do everything for everyone, that mustn't mean that I can't do something for someone. I was once vociferously criticised after a talk I gave by a member of the audience who said that I was squandering money in Bosnia when the need in Africa was so much greater, and any money there would be so much better spent. My answer now is the same as then. I didn't see it is an 'either/or', and the money wasn't mine. The British government had decided to use taxpayer's money to give aid to the former Yugoslavia and in response I put together the best programme I could, based on the needs we had identified. As I said to my critic, I was not given a pot of money and told to go forth and do good. I was instead given an opportunity to help a specific group of people, at a specific time. This hasn't stopped me lobbying for support to countries in Africa, or indeed anywhere where there is a need. But I try to do what I can, where I can, and when I can.

UNDAC was born out of an outpouring of support to Armenia that contrasted sharply with the difficulties encountered in putting to best use all that was being offered. People, organisations and even countries, were giving what they thought most likely to be needed, not what they knew to be needed, and too often, simply what they had. Unsolicited gifts, whether of goods or people, divert the time and attention of those engaged in dealing directly with the disaster. Moreover, without any agreed organised registration and verification process, the authorities in Armenia had to first establish the nature of what was being given and if or how it might be best and safely used. Self-declared 'Rescue Teams', of varying skills and experience, roamed the rubble. One was literally just a man and his dog. He claimed one of the limited places on the plane from Moscow to Leninakan for himself, but remarkably another one for his dog. Two precious places that could have been put to much better use. Medical teams too were of varying quality. Although me and my team had responded to a request for help, we were inexperienced in responding to disasters on such a scale. On my return to the UK I resolved to work with colleagues, both nationally and internationally, to improve the coordination and focus of the international disaster response. The UN looked closely at its own responses too and how it might use its international standing and influence best to work with affected countries to ensure the aid they received was more accurately targeted on the needs they had identified.

So, the United Nations Disaster Assessment and Coordination team was established. Of the twenty original recruits, eighteen of us had been in Armenia. An international pool of experts would now be recruited and trained, and from its ranks, a team dispatched immediately international assistance was requested. Working with the affected government, they would agree and publish the results of a rapid needs assessment, to which those wishing to offer assistance, could refer. The initiative has proven to be remarkably durable and is very active to this day. The advent of the internet has made the results of its assessments even more accessible. Nevertheless, some charities still send their goods and people to disasters, irrespective of what needs have been identified. I have some sympathy for their actions: they genuinely want to help, and to keep their funds coming in, they must be in the public eye. If other charities are there, then they must be there too, or miss out on the funding and publicity opportunities. It is hard to break the vicious cycle and be the first to hold back. That is not to say that help is not required. Even if you don't have the special skills, equipment or experience that are being requested you can still help. You can give money.

The frequent riposte to this is that 'you don't know where the money goes.' 'There is corruption.' 'It will not get to the people who need it most.' All these are valid arguments, but they can be applied equally to the dispatch of goods. Unless you follow your donation continuously from its source to its final recipient, you will not know for sure that it did what you had hoped. If though you give money to a reputable agency – UK-Med, the Red Cross, MSF, or the Disasters Emergency Committee, for example – the degree of scrutiny and governance is such that the money is more likely than not to be well spent. Anyway, that's what I do.

The Boxing Day Asian tsunami of 2004 is a good example of the issues around how best to help after these massive and devastating disasters. My team didn't respond, because at that time we were focused mainly on providing surgical teams, and we knew from all the published evidence that international surgical teams would be unlikely to be needed after a tsunami. Unlike earthquakes where for every person killed, two or three others are severely injured and will require extensive surgical intervention, in a tsunami the opposite is true. For every person out of 10 who survives, the other nine will have perished. As brutal as it sounds, you cannot be severely injured and swim. So, either you escape the tsunami altogether or suffer injuries so minor that you are able to swim and save yourself. So, fewer patients will need surgical operations than after an earthquake, for example, and certainly the affected countries are unlikely to require the services of additional surgical teams from other countries.

And we know that all those unburied dead pose little, if any, serious threat to the physical health of the living – as difficult as that may be to accept and how deeply ingrained it may be in our psyche. The psychological effect of the unburied dead is a different matter altogether. Their swollen appearance and the sweet sickly smell of decay triggers a deep primeval instinct. We all find it abhorrent. It is also so dehumanising to see mothers, fathers, sisters, and brothers cast aside and so brutally exposed. I have seen many dead bodies. I have been in situations where hundreds of dead bodies have lain all around me. I am always disturbed greatly by the sight and the smell, and still at times have to steel myself to carry on. But even more than this is the anguish I feel for the suffering and distress of those who may later have to sift through this appalling detritus in search of their loved ones. That is why mass graves must be avoided if at all possible. There will come a time when they will have to be reopened. I have stood alongside relatives looking at the decomposed faces of those they once held in their arms. As bad as it was for me, it was but nothing compared to the appalling agony they so bravely endured.

I once asked a distinguished senior member of MSF which mission he was most proud of and which mission did he regret. He was most proud of his time in Darfur. To him it epitomised the core values of the organisation. There they were indeed 'doctors without borders', going into Darfur when the Sudanese government was saying they couldn't, and going back again every time they were thrown out. His biggest regret was the Asian tsunami. All his years of experience told him that medical teams such as theirs would not be required, given the nature of the impact on health of a tsunami. However, he said that the pressure to respond from the public and the press became so great that in the end he capitulated. The cries of 'why aren't you there when everybody else is there,' with its implied prejudice and indifference, compelled him in the end to send a team. 'And?', I asked. 'My original view proved to be correct,' he sighed. Reflecting on the response to the tsunami some years later, the head of the Disasters Emergency Committee (DEC) in the UK emphasised that in most cases, 'providing people with training and building materials or cash following a large-scale disaster means that more people can start rebuilding their lives more quickly.'

*

I did several missions for UNDAC, including an assessment mission to Sierra Leone during the 'Blood Diamonds' civil war in 2000, immediately after I had finished my work in Kosovo. This was a particularly sensitive mission as the United Nations Mission in Sierra Leone (UNAMSIL) had been authorised to protect civilians under 'imminent threat of physical violence,' thereby setting it up militarily against the Revolutionary United Front (RUF) and compromising its impartiality and neutrality.[13] This decision brought it into conflict with at least two of the humanitarian principles and consequently compromised any cooperation between itself and humanitarian organisations. There were four of us in the team and my brief was to identify any specific issues related to health. Life expectancy then, as now, was amongst the lowest in the world, with people living in abject poverty. There was little if any health system. By way of example, there was only one trained psychiatrist and three trained gynaecologists for the whole country. In practice many people probably had no effective access to healthcare at all. In the absence of a national health service, the public hospitals and clinics charged for their services. These, the poorest people in the world, simply could not meet the costs.

The main teaching hospital was the Connaught Hospital in Freetown, the capital. There were no medically trained anaesthetic doctors at all, but one nurse anaesthetist who provided anaesthetic services for all 263 beds. MSF were present in the hospital and providing the backbone for the delivery of health services, particularly safe surgery. They also provided food to the hospital, maintained the generator, and provided it with fuel. They ran a ward for the war wounded and carried out surgical operations on war injuries every day. I discovered that local surgeons would only operate for money, and so the penniless were referred to MSF. It was their presence in the country at the time of the ebola outbreak that was instrumental in bringing the plight of its people to the attention of the world and supported them in their recovery. But as in all humanitarian emergencies, it was the profound vulnerability caused by their abject poverty that had already laid down the foundations for the later outbreak of ebola.

The ICRC was also present in Freetown supporting the Princess Christian Maternity Hospital. When I visited, facilities were very basic, worse even than the Connaught Hospital. The Children's Hospital was similarly run down. It was only about half full, which was a gross anomaly given the young age of the Sierra Leonean population and half the population were now living in Freetown. It was obviously a reflection of the fact that, even when your child was desperately sick, you had no access to secondary healthcare if you were poor.

The most disturbing site was the 'Kissy Mental Hospital.' My notes read:

```
the regime is shocking. The most disturbed lie on a
bare concrete floor to which they are permanently
chained, in a building that has no windows and no
sanitation. If/when their behaviour modifies, they
graduate to being chained to a bed in a dirty ward.
Eventually they may graduate to a bed in a
refurbished ward. MSF Holland have done an
```

```
excellent job in refurbishing several wards, but
these are underused for fear of damage by violent
patients. On the other hand, Sierra Leone's only
psychiatrist says he has no or very few
tranquilizers. The patients cannot pay for
medication and are often abandoned by their
families. The staff are mostly untrained. It is
claimed 80% of current admissions are drug induced
psychosis involving marijuana, alcohol, heroin,
ephedrine and gunpowder.
```

I made a firm recommendation for the provision of ample supplies of psychiatric medication.

I also visited facilities for the war wounded amputees. The RUF deliberately amputated limbs as a punishment and a warning to others. I noted that in spite of the large amount of media attention they'd received, the problem was now being contained. One complication of this attention I noted, had been a corresponding resistance on the part of amputees to move out of their special camp for fear of losing the extra assistance and attention brought to them by their notoriety. I saw a steady stream of photojournalists roaming freely to randomly photograph the mutilated, who themselves gladly posed as requested, and showed off their stumps for maximum effect.

I'd found a similar phenomenon earlier that year in Kosovo, when young children with amputations from landmines were fêted by the international press to such an extent that we couldn't get them to use their artificial limbs, get up and walk out of the hospital: they craved the attention. It was only when we banned the press from roaming freely across the hospital, and gave the children the love and care they needed and deserved, that they rapidly adapted to the artificial limbs, abandoned their beds and wheelchairs, and went home. I am not immune from criticism in this regard. When I was in Belgrade at the start of the war I was taken to a hospital for spinal injuries. A young girl, no more than twelve years old perhaps, had been shot through the neck by a sniper and was now paralysed from the neck downwards. I was encouraged by my minder to take a photograph of her to show the world that the Serbs too were victims of atrocities. Somewhat reluctantly I raised my camera and pointed it to this matchstick figure, emotionally passive in a bed far too big for her tiny frame. As I did, she caught my eye, and moved the only muscles she could and smiled. I felt ashamed for intruding on her privacy and shamed further by witnessing her childlike willingness to please, and her desire for attention.

There were up to 1 million displaced persons in Sierra Leone because of the protracted civil war, with 20 per cent of the population living in camps. I noted that the humanitarian community and the government of Sierra Leone discouraged the formation and maintenance of these camps, as any support to them might be perceived as encouragement to stay or encouragement to come when the aim was to resettle people in their communities. However, the ongoing crisis meant that thousands had been in the camps for well over a year and the lack of support had left them in a critical condition. The government of Sierra Leone added to the problem by preventing registration of new entrants. They still arrived, of course, but entered the camps unregistered, and so were not counted in the numbers for feeding and the provision of other resources. An already bad problem was getting worse. This all went into the report and we made our way home.

On the plane travelling out to Sierra Leone I got into conversation with my new colleagues, one of whom told me that he had just retired from the British army. When I'd asked him if he had ever been to Sierra Leone before he told me that he'd been there only the year before while serving in the army. I automatically asked him about a story I'd seen of British officers who had been held hostage, and to my amazement he said that he had been one of them: held captive in the jungle by a rebel group known as the Armed Forces Revolutionary Council, and now going back voluntarily into a still very unstable situation. A quite remarkable man, and another example of the many acts of quiet courage that I've been privileged to witness.

The journey into Sierra Leone was also memorable for other reasons. Because of the war in Sierra Leone there were no direct flights and so we had to first fly to Conakry in Guinea from where the UN operated a daily helicopter service into Freetown Sierra Leone for its staff. You checked in at a wooden hut on the edge of a field where an ageing Russian helicopter (similar to the one in which I might have died a year or two later) was waiting to whisk you over the jungle and into the capital of the neighbouring country. On boarding the helicopter, you were given a clipboard in which you essentially signed your life away. It stated that the UN bore no responsibility for you should anything untoward happen. Having come this far I simply decided to sign. More worrying still was the information they gave us that the rebels had expressed an intention to shoot down helicopters now that the UN appeared to be party to the conflict. The good news, they said without irony, is that we know they only have one surface-to-air missile, and looking at the passenger list for today, we don't see anyone here that they would be likely to consider worth expending it upon. So off we set, flying very low, skimming the treetops of the jungle, with the crew looking out for any untoward activity below.

I struck up a conversation with a young woman sat opposite me who seemed particularly nervous. I tried to reassure her as best I could, although there comes a point when you just must face up to the risks you are taking. She told me that this was her first mission, which explained her anxiety, and that she had been sent by a very small independent charity to set up a 'creative play programme' for the children in Sierra Leone. On this her first mission, she was travelling alone. She had never been in an insecure environment before, let alone a war. On landing in a similar field in Sierra Leone we were taken in UN vehicles to a somewhat rundown hotel on the edge of the city. Brooding militia, all brandishing AK-47s, were loitering around the hotel entrance and throughout the lobby. She was clearly upset and frightened by their presence, and immediately on receiving her key, took herself to her room and locked herself in. You could hear gunfire outside, but I felt relatively secure within the hotel. It had clearly seen better days and not all the rooms were functioning, but it was adequate. There was even a television set, that with judicious manipulation of the aerial and avoidance of a large rat that had made its home behind it, allowed a group of us that evening to watch a snowy vision of a football match. But she was nowhere to be seen. She did not appear for dinner nor breakfast in the morning. We set off early to begin our work and I learned on my return that evening that she had never ventured out of her room until the UN helicopter was due to head back to Conakry which she duly reboarded and went home. I felt enormous sympathy for her and the courage she had shown by volunteering for this mission and making it as far as the country. She was also brave enough to acknowledge to herself that she couldn't cope with the uncertainty and threat that now surrounded her, and so withdrew. I do not have much sympathy, though, for the organisation that allowed this woman to go into such a dangerous environment with no preparation or support. This, and a thousand other examples of inadequate preparation and training has fuelled my desire, and those of my colleagues, to strengthen the international response to humanitarian crises.

*

Whilst working in and out of Bosnia I also did another mission for the United Nations Disaster Assessment and Coordination (UNDAC) Team, and travelled to Cape Verde in April 1995 – before it became a tourist attraction – in order to assess the impact of a volcanic eruption on Fogo, one of its smaller islands. The volcano had last erupted in the year of my birth, 1951, following which several thousand people had returned and scratched a living from farming in the large basin around the cone that had formed after the eruption. We flew from Geneva, via Lisbon, into Praia, the capital of Cape Verde, and then by light aircraft to the island of Fogo, where the only place for the plane to land was on the beach. The volcano was still active, and the fear was that if it stayed active at the current level, the lava flow would reach the remaining inhabitants. When the volcano erupted it opened a vent in the side of the 1951 cone and lava was flowing up to 20 m/h. I witnessed this for myself, when I went to take a closer look and got closer than I'd intended. I could hear the rumble of the eruption but as I turned around the side of the cone, I suddenly felt the heat blast and the noise of what sounded like several jet engines. I was stopped in my tracks but snapped out of it when I realised the earth around me was moving as rocks were being pushed by an approaching flow of lava.

One of the issues we highlighted was that there was already an unrelated cholera outbreak on the main island of Sao Tiago, and considered it only a question of time before it spread to Fogo where it would spread rapidly amongst people living in tented camps having been displaced by the eruption. As is usually the case, it is not the incident itself that causes the outbreak of disease, but rather the following mass movement of people into unsatisfactory and insanitary conditions. Sometimes the incident, such as the earth-quake in Haiti, precipitates the mass movement of people into the country, and it is they who bring with them the disease – like the cholera from UN troops in the case of Haiti.

The health services in Cape Verde were struggling to contain the cholera outbreak, largely due to a shortage of trained healthcare staff. The report we produced was circulated widely, but on my return to the UK, I also forwarded it directly to the Overseas Development Administration with a request for funding for me to send a team to work in support of the healthcare workers in Cape Verde. I followed it up with a phone call, and while appearing sympathetic to the needs of the people I was describing, the person on the other end of the phone said words to the effect of 'Cape Verde, that's not ours is it? I'm pretty sure that's Portugal's.' The days of Empire were not quite over it seemed, and I asked him if he would like to be quoted on that. After a pause he replied, 'not espe-cially', and after a short but fruitful discussion, he said the application would be approved. And so it was. We sent nurses and doctors to Fogo for almost a year after the eruption to work in support of the local health care staff to successfully contain the cholera outbreak and stay until it had gone. An important principle that I have worked hard to establish is that the emergency response can, and often should, be the starter for a more prolonged engagement that can help a vulnerable community get back on its feet and 'build back better'.

As well as UNDAC, the International Search and Rescue Advisory Group, INSARAG, was created following the experiences of Armenia. International standards would be established, and a system of registration, accreditation and reaccreditation would be developed. These important developments predated those that would follow in respect of medical teams, and in many ways set the template for what would become the WHO Emergency Medical Teams Initiative. There is a certain irony here. The impact of international search and rescue teams on saving lives is in practice very small. That is not because of any lack of skill; far from it. It is simply that the window of opportunity to save lives after earthquakes in particular is surprisingly small, and although there are always exceptions, most of those who are rescued after earthquakes are rescued by fellow survivors. The remainder are rescued by local and national rescue teams. But the teams that have to cross continents and oceans to get there will simply arrive too late. To illustrate this, I tell my students that should the building in which we are in suddenly collapse upon us all, we will not be lying in the rubble waiting for a team from Nepal to come and rescue us. That is not to say there are no other things that international search and rescue teams can do to help; the UK International Search and Rescue (ISAR) team helped greatly in Nepal by reinforcing buildings and providing logistical support to the UK Emergency Medical Team.

Only a year after the terrible Boxing Day tsunami a devastating earthquake shook Kashmir. An extensive national and international humanitarian response was mounted and many of the widespread Pakistani diaspora went there to help. Amongst these were a small group of doctors I got to know and whose families were of Pakistani origin. Like my experience almost twenty years before, they were overwhelmed by the enormity of what they saw and concerned about their, and others' preparation and training. They contacted the Royal College of Emergency Medicine to seek advice and were referred on to me. By then I was recovering from my heavy metal poisoning but not yet back to full-time work, and UK-Med had been dormant during the time of my most serious illness. We discussed the best step forwards and I advised them how to establish themselves as a charity and a non-governmental organisation (NGO). However, after a lengthy discussion they said they preferred to work through UK-Med, which in effect rebooted the organisation after my enforced period of withdrawal. A few months after the earthquake I joined them on a follow-up mission to Pakistan.

*

In 2008, a massive earthquake struck Sichuan in the south west of China. At first, I did not consider there would be a role for what was still quite a small team. However, unbeknown to me, the UK ambassador to the UN had held talks with his Chinese counterpart, running on the lines of 'if the UK were to offer aid would it be accepted?'; and 'if China were to request assistance would it be given?' The upshot was, I was asked by the Foreign & Commonwealth Office to lead a team to the epicentre of the earthquake.

Our mission to China threw up a number of issues. China is a powerful country with huge resources, and did not especially need assistance from the UK. In particular it was not waiting to be rescued by a small band of UK healthcare professionals. The UK, though, does not offer help to every country, and China is very selective in from where and from whom it accepts support. Although nothing was said specifically, I appreciated that both the offer and its acceptance were playing out on a wider diplomatic stage. So, what to do? We were back in the realm of gesture. But I have found gestures can be powerful and find myself usually more concerned about empty gestures than gestures alone. There would seem to me some good to be done in responding to this request, and further good to do by avoiding the harm of a rejection. But of course, in dealing with China there are always the significant concerns that surround their human rights record to confront, and by responding to this humanitarian emergency, were we also compromising other values? However limited our assistance might prove to be on this occasion, there were fellow human beings in severe distress and whose government had asked for our assistance. I have also always been drawn more to engagement than isolation. I said yes.

There followed some email traffic between Manchester, London, and Beijing. The FCO would fund all our expenses, although we as a team would all be volunteers, seconded from the NHS. Before leaving we emailed our CVs to Beijing and almost by return received letters of authorisation to practice medicine in China for '30 days from the date of this email.' We flew to Beijing, where we changed planes for Chengdu and were met on arrival by British and Chinese officials. From there we were transported to Mian Yang, the nearest city to the epicentre. There was considerable damage to buildings, but it was functioning, and the hospital was working. Our presence seemed to cause something of a stir, as this was not a tourist area, but it was a welcome.

We were put up in a small hotel near to the hospital. The building had clearly suffered some damage but most of the floors were still open for business. A translator-cum-minder was allocated to us and we set off for the hospital, where we began work immediately. There were many crush injuries, as we expected, and the surgical team worked alongside the Chinese surgical teams to perform limb salvage surgery with the aim of avoiding amputations.

Just as there is an enduring myth about the risk to the living from the unburied dead after earthquakes, so there is a similar myth among some medical practitioners that crushed limbs must always be amputated immediately. Certainly, if major complications have already been established, then an amputation may be inevitable. But the consequences of amputation for those already struggling in poverty, in an environment where rehabilitation and prostheses are limited or non-existent, can be devastating. You must do all you can to preserve as much of the limb as you can. But what if a person is trapped by the limb and can only be released by its amputation. This is a scenario common in films, but uncommon in my long clinical experience. I have completed a limb amputation when someone was trapped under a train, but this was merely to cut through the final few centimetres of flesh – the train having done the rest. Traumatic amputations like this produce what are termed 'guillotine' amputations for obvious reasons and the term is also used for any emergency amputation where speed is of the essence. However, a competent surgeon will then refashion the stump to ensure that bone and muscle are covered by skin. Sadly, in the many earthquakes that I have attended I have seen too many people left in their beds with a limb severed completely through and an open stump weeping into bloodied bandages. My colleagues and I have worked for many years with the World Health Organisation and the Red Cross to improve the approach to amputations and emergencies and I'm pleased to say that these efforts have borne fruit in recent years. Sadly, in China one of the first patients we saw was a young teenage girl who had a guillotine amputation through the middle of her right upper leg, with no attempt having been made to surgically cover the raw, exposed flesh and bone of her thigh. Our plastic surgeon, Mr. Waseem Saeed, safely closed the wound, which when healed allowed a prosthesis to be fitted.

Waseem and I were operating on another case, on the thirteenth floor of the surgical building, when a 6.4 magnitude aftershock struck. It had been heralded by a short-lived, much weaker, shaking of the building which had alarmed me, but not to the point of abandoning the surgical list for the day. However midway through the operation the table began to move violently. The instruments bounced off their tray and fell to the floor. The ceiling of the operating theatre rippled so badly that the operating light that was firmly fixed to it swayed backwards and forwards over our heads. We couldn't see through the windows as the glass vibrated so violently it appeared frosted. The Chinese nurses in the operating theatre screamed: they had survived the original earthquake and their nerves were stretched to the limit. We leaned forwards over our sleeping patient and held onto him, lest he fall from the operating table onto the floor. The shaking got even more violent and seemed to me to last forever. Just as I began to think 'so this is how it ends' it stopped, as suddenly as it had begun.

An eerie silence fell upon us, followed by anxious whispering, and a rapid animated discussion about how we would get our patient and ourselves down the thirteen floors to safety. We found a stretcher and carefully slid the sleeping patient onto it and then slowly moved him step-by-step, floor by floor, down to the ground floor, hoping all the time that no further aftershocks were imminent. All the while the anaesthetist kept our blissfully ignorant patient asleep. He lay at a 45-degree angle on the stairs and we had to hold onto him to keep him on the stretcher. When we finally got to safety outside, we found that everyone had evacuated the building and was working out of tents in the hospital grounds. We took our patient into one of these, placed him on a temporary operating table, where Mr. Saeed could finally complete his operation. Aftershocks continued at regular intervals, and the already tense atmosphere in the city reached a palpable level of anxiety. Not only were the already damaged buildings at risk of finally toppling if there were any further significant quakes, but post-earthquake landslides in the mountains immediately above the city had led to the build-up of huge amounts of water behind them, and the creation of new 'quake lakes'. If a further severe aftershock, or even the sheer weight of water, caused a breach in their walls, then the city would be drowned in an avalanche of mud and water, and all of its occupants, including ourselves, doomed to perish in the slurry. As we carried on with our work in the hospital, we could see the city being steadily evacuated. We watched the television news in awe as the People's Liberation Army (PLA) climbed the treacherous mountain, and by sheer weight of numbers, shored up the walls of the 'quake lakes'. Just when we thought catastrophe was about to be averted, the reinforcements failed, and they had to begin again.

The epicentre had been cordoned off by the army, with only permitted vehicles allowed into the area, and not before the wheels of their vehicles had been sprayed with some unknown chemical and the occupants had dipped their hands and feet into bowls of what appeared to be something similar. We too were subjected to this ritual, which was as dramatic in its theatrical show of apparent disease control as it was ineffective. We were joined in Mian Yang by a senior public health official from Beijing, with whom I had a very illuminating discussion about addressing people's fears in the middle of an emergency. He candidly said that he knew that me, like he, knew that spraying the vehicles and dipping our hands and feet in bowls of an unknown fluid would do little, if anything, to control infection, but it would go a long way to control the fear of infection.

He asked me to address a public meeting in the city. He said there was an unjustified but alarming fear of disease from the many unburied dead. In spite of the government's best efforts, anxiety was only growing. There was an additional fear of plague breaking out in the region, which custom and practice believed to be released into the community after an earthquake. Plague was endemic in the region, so a not altogether totally unfounded association. The aim of my address was to allay their fears of epidemics. 'But why me?' I asked. 'Because you're a foreigner, they'll believe you.' And so I addressed an open-air public meeting, through an interpreter, and did my best to explain that earthquakes were not followed by epidemics, and that if people boiled water before drinking and paid great attention to personal hygiene, the risk of illness would be significantly reduced. After my talk I was approached by a nurse who asked one of the most heart-breaking and morally stretching questions I have ever received: 'If you find yourself in a hospital ward with your patients when the earthquake strikes, do you stay with your patient or run?' I didn't ask what she had done, but the anguish in her face told me. I said 'You can only do what you think is right at the time.' She was as disappointed with my answer as I was.

As time went on, and just as in Armenia many years before when the bulk of the work shifted from Leninakan to the capital Yerevan, we moved our centre of operations to Chengdu, the capital of Sichuan province. There we continue to work with Chinese nurses and doctors and established solid professional and personal relationships that have endured to this day.

A special feature of earthquakes in modern cities lies in the consequences of living in high-rise buildings. Opportunities for escape are limited and many are killed or severely injured in the crush. Horrifically, many choose to jump rather than await the collapse of the building. There are therefore large numbers of spinal injuries amongst those who survive. We recognised this, along with the almost non-existent provision of specialist spinal injury rehabilitation units. On my return to the UK I successfully applied for funding to support a two-year spinal injury rehabilitation programme that saw specialists from the UK work with colleagues in China to facilitate the management of paralysed patients in their homes. A particular highlight was witnessing a young occupational therapist demonstrate how to get in and out of a car independently. She had been addressing a large number of young people, each paralysed below the waist, and in attendance with their parent. The law in China had just been changed to allow those with paraplegia to independently drive a specially adapted car. 'What good is that to me?' said a young man. 'I want to be independent and go out without my mother', at which the audience giggled, 'but I still need her with me to help me in and out of the car and to stow my wheelchair.' She tried to reassure them that there were ways this could be done, but he was singularly unconvinced. So, she asked him to show her his car. We all left the auditorium and followed her to the car park, where she showed him exactly how to align himself alongside the car, slide himself across onto his seat, collapse the wheelchair, and place it in the car behind his seat. And reverse the process to get out. All unattended. I thought he was going to cry, and the crowd around him applauded. As a *pièce de résistance* she then made him do it again while she videoed the whole procedure and gave him a copy of the DVD to take home. We later reprinted one for every person who had attended her lecture and then some for the hospital. I think of this as one of the most powerful and cost-effective interventions I've been privileged to witness. It is not always the glamorous and the swashbuckling that do the most good. I have seen the quiet work of rehabilitation specialists transforming lives around the world, often in the most austere of circumstances, and for long after we, the emergency teams, have left. As we developed our national EMT, we ensured that rehabilitation specialists are core members of the team from the moment they land in country.

My work in the earthquake in China helped me establish a long and fruitful working relationship with medical and nursing colleagues there, which has endured to this day. In the UK we are fortunate to live in a part of the world that is spared many of the world's most violent environmental hazards, with most earthquakes, tsunamis, typhoons etc., occurring many thousands of miles away. However strong our willingness is to help others, we in the UK will always be far away from the centre of some of the biggest disasters. It is therefore imperative that those affected countries and their close neighbours have the resources to respond. Through my work with the World Health Organisation, and following on from my work in the Wenchuan earthquake, I have supported the development of China's, and other countries', International Emergency Medical Teams, and seen them take a leading role in disaster relief in the most vulnerable parts of the world. I look forward to the time when international humanitarian relief no longer needs to cross oceans to reach the most needy, but will be a gift from their neighbours.

*

Ten years after the earthquake I was invited to attend a memorial ceremony for the victims of the earthquake. I was proud to stand in the grounds of the hospital in Mian Yang alongside Chinese colleagues who I had worked with at the time, to honour the memory of the dead and give thanks for those who had survived. There is a mural depicting the events of the earthquake in the entrance to the hospital that extends all the way down the main corridor. Featured in it are photographs of the UK-Med team. In a show of solidarity and friendship with mainland China, after the Wenchuan earthquake, the people of Hong Kong raised millions in disaster relief, and supported many programmes in the earthquake-stricken area. This culminated in the Hong Kong Jockey Club funding a new Institute for Disaster Management and Reconstruction in Chengdu, where I am currently Visiting Professor of Disaster Medicine. I can only hope that the goodwill I know exists between the peoples of the mainland and the island can once again be allowed to flourish.

10.

Disaster Tourism

Haiti

There were many improvements in the international disaster response that came out of the earthquake in Armenia. But still ill-prepared, ill-equipped, and inexperienced teams and individuals continue to pour into disaster-stricken areas. Their intentions may have been good, but if uninvited and, worse still, unprepared – dependent on others for food, shelter and supplies – they are more likely than not to add to the troubles of the affected country. And any problem of this type, even if only amongst a small percentage of those who responded, is still likely to be a bigger problem, given the scale of the aid industry now. There are 10 million NGOs worldwide. On the one hand this can be considered testimony to the human spirit and its desire to help those in need, but on the other, this outpouring of altruism needs for me always to be matched with a corresponding professionalism, whereby those who deliver aid do so to a recognised standard and with the same level of accountability they would expect for themselves and their family from anyone ministering to their needs. Above all any response must be doing something in response to an expressed need and a clear invitation.

There are some who harbour concerns about the use of the word 'professionalism' in this context, with its implication of it being a job like any other, and perhaps even a job that attracts a high salary. This is not how it is generally meant to be understood, although I agree some 'charities' do seem to lay themselves open to criticism for the scale of the salaries they pay their executive staff. Rather, it is meant to emphasise that even when the circumstances in which you are working are highly abnormal, and at times difficult and even dangerous, standards still need to be applied. I too often hear it argued that standards cannot be maintained to the highest level when the circumstances are so insecure and unstable, but it is in precisely in these circumstances that we must try our hardest. Even more concerning is the argument that when local standards are poor, we can dial ours down accordingly. Local standards, if indeed they are poor, are usually that way because the people themselves are poor, and simply lack the resources to do things in a way they would want. We must all work together, despite the obvious and many difficulties, to achieve and maintain the standards we all deserve.

The unregulated free-for-all that has been allowed to go unchecked in too many humanitarian responses has been fertile ground for the growth of the abuses that have come to light in recent years. But perhaps my greatest concern relates to a certain type of medical assistance given to poorer countries. I have encountered doctors who enjoy working in humanitarian emergencies, or on 'medical missions' overseas, precisely because of a lack of regulation and accountability – I still do. Worse still, they value it for the opportunity to carry out procedures for which they are neither licensed nor trained in their own country. This phenomenon can also be seen in the approach by some to the overseas medical student elective. When I was a medical student some fifty years ago, students would boast of the unsupervised surgery they did in a poor country, far away from the supervision of the University and the General Medical Council. If challenged, the mantra of 'any help is better than no help' was always trotted out. Played like a trump card, it usually ended the discussion. But within medicine of all places, any help cannot always be better than no help. Inexpert help can, and will, do irreparable, and even fatal harm. At the root of it all is an uncritical approach to doing overseas what you could never do at home. Overseas deployment might be seen as a way of gaining experience rapidly and without responsibility for the consequences of your inevitable mistakes. I had hoped such attitudes would fade with more enlightened medical practice, but talking to medical students now, I have my doubts that it has gone away completely. Moreover, it is still alive in those established in their career. 'Practicing medicine in its purest form' without the burdensome 'unnecessary paperwork', I've heard them say. But if we are not to be hiding imperialism, or rank racism, behind a thin veil of apparent altruism, then we must adhere to the same standards and regulations we look to for ourselves and our own, wherever we practice. For a start, we must be authorised to practice in that country, something that has been too often overlooked. We must be fully insured. Whilst we live in fear of the thud of the solicitor's letter dropping through the letterbox onto the mat, patients have a right of redress if they have been harmed through our negligence or misconduct. This applies everywhere. There may be obvious mitigating circumstances when working in the most austere of conditions, but you remain accountable to your patient.

*

This phenomenon of rich doctors dispensing largesse to poor patients, without any true accountability, rumbles on in any number of 'medical missions', but probably reached its zenith, or should that be nadir, in 2010 during the medical response to the earthquake in Haiti. An event to be subsequently described in the medical literature as 'disaster tourism' and 'a medical shame'. As the scale of the disaster rapidly unfolded, with ultimately over 200,000 Haitians thought to have been killed and over 1 million people displaced from their homes, the Department for International Development of the UK government quickly put together a large-scale response. Working with the logistical support of British NGO Medical Emergency Relief International (MERLIN), I led a specialist limb salvage surgical team, drawn from UK-Med. By rotating staff, mainly seconded from the NHS, we were able to provide a continuous surgical service for three months after the earthquake.

I travelled with the forward team into the Dominican Republic and from there overland into Haiti. The airport in the capital, Port-au-Prince, had been damaged and was only accepting a small number of relief flights at that time, with as yet no passenger service. Nevertheless, John Travolta did somehow manage to fly his own plane into Port-au-Prince, from where he distributed food and blankets, I understand, bringing with him several hundred Scientologists to carry out 'healing by touch'. I witnessed these practitioners in their orange T-shirts walking in groups through the streets of the city, but have to report that I found no evidence of any miraculous tactile recoveries. I also saw voodoo practised by the relatives of patients lying in our hospital beds, flapping cockerels held over them by their legs, women spraying water from their mouths into their faces – but at least they were also getting antibiotics.

We registered with the UN and the Ministry of Health looked for a suitable safe place to establish our field hospital. One of the team found what had been a tennis court at some time in the past and which provided a good flat hardstanding with a high perimeter wall. We also found in the grounds of a hotel a safe place to establish our living quarters and pitch our tents. We made sure that our tents were placed well away from buildings that might topple upon them with any aftershock. It proved to be a good choice. There was running water from the showers next to the disused swimming pool, and when a significant after-shock did strike one early morning, other than feeling the earth sway up and down and side to side beneath me as I was sliding out of my small one-man tent, I knew I was in no danger. It is not earthquakes themselves that kill people, but falling buildings. Our choice of location was also reinforced by seeing the occupants of the hotel itself running for their lives as the building shook violently. We would not in fairness have chosen to stay in the hotel, given the risk of aftershocks, but our choice was limited in that it had already been occupied by journalists who, whilst expressing embarrassment at seeing the medical team sleeping in one-man tents on the floor outside, admitted also that they were not embarrassed enough to swap.

We quickly established a routine of early morning ward rounds, daily operating lists and outpatient/emergency clinics. We recruited local staff and invited other NGOs already working in Haiti to join us. We established a particularly fruitful relationship with the Irish NGO, GOAL, who essentially ran the emergency department of our field hospital. There was also a US fundamentalist Christian medical missionary group, already working in Haiti when the earthquake struck and destroyed their building, who joined us in what became a consortium. They had many fine nurses and doctors in their group and a particularly active group of young volunteers who made an exceptional contribution to the hospital. They built a range of shelters seemingly out of nothing, along with a building for our sterilisation unit. But there were some notable exceptions in their midst, reflecting a darker side to either their religious beliefs or the broader culture from which they had emerged, or possibly both. By this, I mean a tendency to treat the Haitians as 'other', and so different to them that they did not seem to warrant the same standard of care as they would give their own.

There were many burned children in Haiti. The poor lived in shacks heated and lit by open fires. Children left unattended while their parents worked to keep them from starvation fell into these fires. When the earthquake struck these fires also set fire to the shacks in which they lived. Just as in Kurdistan many years before, we had to treat burned children forced to live too close to open flames. Changing burns dressings in anyone, but particularly in children, can be an extremely painful and distressing procedure. The misery can be alleviated by adequate pain relief, and if necessary, general anaesthesia. But I was horrified one morning when, following the screams of a small infant to their source, I found a member of this Christian group bedecked in their antiquated costume, ripping the burns dressings from the raw burned skin of an infant, gripped tightly to prevent them from thrashing about. My shouts for her to stop joined the screams of the child in pain until she stopped what she was doing, and the child's screams slowed into hiccups and sobs. 'What on earth do you think you are you doing?' I bellowed. With a look of utter distain, she told me she was simply changing the child's dressing. 'But we do that with pain relief or anaesthesia,' I said. '*We* always do it this way', was her reply, 'and anyway it will be over in a minute.' 'We don't do it this way in my hospital,' I said bluntly. 'We have more than enough pain medicine to give the child, and anaesthetists who can put her to sleep if that is not enough,' I explained. 'We do not allow children to suffer in this way.' With a look of superiority and utter distain I hadn't seen since confronted by the pharmacist in Failsworth almost a lifetime before, she said, 'but they don't feel pain like we do.' I rescued the child from her clutches, and from then on, her dressings were changed with full pain relief. I spoke to the leader of the religious group and explained in no uncertain terms that if they wished to continue working with us, they were working to our protocols, and with the exception of that particular nurse who we never saw again, they adapted and did a lot of good work.

*

There were hundreds, perhaps thousands, of unburied dead in Haiti. I understood the profound terror their physical presence invoked in an already traumatised population, and corresponding fear of disease they brought. It was over twenty years since I had been in Armenia, but once again in a town square in Haiti, I still felt that same sense of panic wash over me and my breathing quicken, just as when you plunge into the cold sea. I smelt the same sickly scent of decomposition, saw bodies piled head-high all around me. I knew that if I took control of my breathing, slowed it down, and closed my eyes for a moment, the panic would ease and then pass. Mercifully, it did.

One morning a BBC journalist came to the field hospital and asked me for my views on the burgeoning epidemic in Haiti. I asked her to give me some background as to her concerns and she said that the Ministry of Health was now reporting an increase in the recorded numbers of infectious diseases. I explained to her epidemics do not as such directly follow an earthquake, but she was sceptical, and was up against a deadline to get her story onto the evening news. I said that I expected the rise in recorded numbers to be a reflection of a much more accurate monitoring of infectious disease in the population, now that the UN, and in particular the Pan American Health Organisation (PAHO, the equivalent of WHO in the Americas) was present in large numbers. Although the numbers had increased against what was reported before the earthquake, what was being reported now, I suggested, was more likely an accurate reflection of the background presence of endemic infectious disease in this very poor community. 'But how will I know if you are right?', she asked. 'The figures will be roughly the same next week,' I replied. She understood my argument and was prepared to delay her story for a week but added 'I still need a story for the 6 o'clock news.' This gave me my opening to shed a light on another common disaster myth: that amputations will be plentiful and unavoidable. I explained to her how my experience over the years and that of many others, was that badly crushed limbs can often be salvaged, either in part or in whole, and much more often than one might expect. It was, I explained, why we had established this specialist ortho plastic surgical team (a combination of ortho-paedic surgeons working with plastic/reconstructive surgeons) now working in the field hospital. She ran a very good piece that evening on the difficult issues for both doctor and patient that surround emergency amputation, and the following week confirmed my hypothesis on infectious diseases was correct.

There is a dilemma around amputation after limbs are crushed. Judging exactly how damaged the limb is, and particularly if damaged beyond any sort of repair, is difficult in the early stages and there is obvious value in waiting to see what degree of recovery can be achieved. The danger in this is that the crushed tissues, and in particular crushed muscle, might release their contents into the bloodstream, and the large molecules from broken down muscle in particular will clog up the kidneys and lead to kidney failure and ultimately death. Damaged and contaminated tissue is also ripe for infection which if left unchecked will lead to septicaemia and death. Amputate too soon and a person living in poverty will now have the added burden of trying to survive as an amputee, with all the stigma and lack of employment opportunity that can follow. Of course, amputate too late, and even the limited opportunities of an amputee will have been denied to your patient. There is a middle ground to be occupied by experienced surgeons, familiar with earthquake injuries, who will do their best to salvage either the limb itself or as much of its length as possible, and who also know when it's time to bring matters to a close and amputate. Over the years many of us have come together to learn from each other's experiences, run training courses, and encourage surgeons to deploy within well-established organisations to bring the best of care and the greatest chance of a good recovery to some of the most vulnerable people in the world.

In Haiti, though, surgeons from around the world set to work with too few having experience of the type of injuries they found themselves facing, and little or no knowledge of large-scale disaster relief. Had they been better prepared they might have known that while *they* didn't know what they were doing, there were teams in country who did. But they either did not know how to contact the UN coordination centre, or simply refused to do so. Within that centre is an established 'cluster' system, with the 'health cluster' headed up by WHO. There you will find which teams are in country and the services they can offer. I vividly remember a young doctor, still in training though not as a surgeon, who had travelled to Haiti with two companions. He confided to me that he had had to amputate the thumb, index and middle fingers of a young girl, and how awful such a decision was to make, and how terrible he felt for the girl's future. The way he spoke suggested that he was expecting me to be impressed by the gravity of the responsibilities he'd taken upon himself, and to be sympathetic for the terrible decision he'd had to make. 'Why didn't you refer her to a plastic surgeon?' I asked. He looked at me incredulously, almost laughing. I informed him that there were many plastic and reconstructive surgeons now in Haiti, including those in my own team. He fell silent and I spared him my thoughts on how a specialist might have been able to salvage her hand, or at least her all-important thumb. But of course, he had never been to a disaster before: he had seen it on the television and with two of his friends booked a flight to the Dominican Republic and a taxi into Port-au-Prince.

It wasn't just the young and inexperienced who saw Haiti as a surgical playground. A well-known professor of surgery from Europe wrote publicly about how he had arrived in Haiti alone and without any equipment and took it upon himself to amputate a limb with his Swiss Army knife. Without sterility, without pain relief, and I worry without permission. And this wasn't the worst abuse of medical power that I witnessed. An international team was carrying out guillotine amputations without any attempt to fashion any sort of stump, leaving their patients lying alone on the floor after surgery, still anaesthetised, with the bloody stump raw and oozing into filthy bandages. So shocked was I by all that I'd seen I secured funding for a research team to go back into Haiti three months after the acute emergency had subsided. They reviewed records at a rehabilitation centre and interviewed survivors in the local language. They found that the amputation rates for well-known, experienced surgical teams, were similar, and below 10 per cent (in line with published rates from previous earthquakes). The inexperienced teams had amputation rates of over 45 per cent, and the team whose patients I saw lying on the floor had an amputation rate of over 80 per cent. It is possible there may be good reasons for such a startling difference, but only the experienced teams with their low amputation rates kept medical records that could explain, and importantly justify, their actions. The other teams made no medical records and the patients disclosed that they had given no consent to what was carried out. They only knew the doctors were 'foreign'. It is clear to me that too many amputations were done, either too soon or without justification, reflecting a gross lack of experience and understanding of the condition they were treating. In any other circumstance it would be regarded as malpractice. How such abuses can be carried out in full view and with impunity reflects an underlying attitude of 'any help is better than no help', and even worse 'beggars can't be choosers' and 'they should be grateful for what they get.' When the help being offered is surgery offered by someone not trained in that surgical procedure, or worse still by someone not trained in surgery at all, then that is certainly not better than no help at all. All these scenarios were played out in Haiti.

As medical team leader I looked to establish networks with other facilities, particularly Haitian hospitals, and visited a large hospital in the centre of town. To my surprise I found it occupied completely by North American physicians and nurses, all busily running around in their blue scrubs. At the entrance was a large piece of white paper stuck with tape to the wall. It asked you simply to write your name and your specialty. No reference to verification of your qualifications, and certainly no reference to registering with the Ministry of Health to gain authorisation to practice in Haiti. Sadly, such disregard for the basics of medical registration and accountability when working in disasters, particularly in poor countries, was not altogether uncommon at that time, but nevertheless completely unjustified. Such abuse of power would not happen when responding to emergencies in a strong, rich country. Such countries control their borders, whereas we drove into Haiti with only a cursory glance at our passport at the ramshackle border post. Rich countries do not allow anyone in to practice medicine: only if they are needed, and only after their qualifications have been verified and they have been given formal authorisation to practice. We voluntarily registered with the Ministry of Health in Haiti, but there was no overt obligation to do so, and doctors and nurses just turned up and began to work. Nevertheless, the responsibility lies first with us as practitioners, and we shouldn't have to be asked to make ourselves accountable to our patients – wherever we work.

Eventually I found the Haitian hospital staff huddled together in a small room on the top floor of the building. They looked to me to have abandoned all hope of controlling the hospital and had an air of weariness and despondency about them. They were gracious and clearly grateful for the help being provided, as they had neither the manpower nor the resources to cope with a disaster of this magnitude, and probably not even to cope on a day-to-day basis in any event. But there was an atmosphere too of humiliation, of being side-lined in their own hospital. It would have taken very little extra to have engaged them more fully in the work these essentially goodhearted volunteers were doing. I wish they had.

*

A recurring issue for surgical teams in sudden-onset disasters is the provision of oxygen. We try and do as many of our procedures under local anaesthesia, regional blocks (freezing the nerve to a whole limb) or spinal anaesthesia. But some procedures can only be done under general anaesthesia which requires the patient to be given additional oxygen while their breathing is potentially compromised. Transporting oxygen is very difficult as the cylinders are heavy and take up much space on an aircraft. Also, there are very specific aviation rules about the transport of highly inflammable oxygen. For practical reasons, teams rarely travel with their own oxygen, but look for supplies when they arrive in-country. Through a circuitous route I found out that the Brazilian army, who were already in Haiti at the time of the earthquake as part of the UN force, had a large supply of oxygen in huge cylinders stored on a trailer. I made my way to their camp and met with their senior medical officers. Whilst they were using the oxygen for surgical procedures, they had more than enough to meet their needs. They had been treating victims of the earthquake who now needed further specialist reconstructive surgery. We did a deal. Each day we would bring an empty oxygen cylinder to the camp for filling and take it back with us, accompanied by any patients that needed the services of our plastic surgeons. It was an arrangement that worked well and lasted for the duration of our mission.

As the relief effort gathered pace, facilities for establishing a more normal practice improved. PAHO established a blood transfusion service, for example. The *USNS Comfort*, a US hospital ship, arrived offshore, and I was pleasantly surprised one morning to receive an email from one of her medical officers offering assistance. They had specialist blood products that I knew would be of particular benefit to one of our patients. I followed this up with a phone call to the ship where it was agreed they would be transferred to our nearest 'El Zee'. Two countries divided by a common language was never truer. I had no idea what he was talking about but hoped all would eventually become clear. The follow-up email saw 'Zee' become my 'Zed' and LZ emerged from the cloud as Landing Zone. I would pick it up from the main airport, and blood products duly arrived within an hour or so of my request. The patient did very well.

Running an operating theatre in a tent, and running it safely, is a heavy responsibility and one that is carried ultimately by the nurse in charge of the operating theatre. We were blessed with Flora, one of the best in the business. Calm, authoritative, and a match for any misplaced surgical ego. She kept the operating theatre scrupulously clean with a very strict regime of who and when they could enter. She was also a wonderful singer and one night as we sat around the fire our conversation drifted onto folk music. I said that one of my favourite Scottish folk songs was the 'Mingulay Boat Song'. She told me that her grandparents were amongst the last to leave the island in 1912, after which it became uninhabited. We sang the Mingulay Boat Song together, in two-part harmony. Our voices floated out into the coal black night as the whole camp fell still and listened.

I have many such memories of warmth and pleasure that emerged from the ruins of disaster. It is not all doom and gloom. People do recover. I was walking towards my apartment in Sarajevo once, having just dealt with some of the most appalling injuries I'd yet seen, when through the open window came the tune of 'Fields of Gold', played on a small tape player recently purchased by a team member. It was a glorious sunny afternoon, a golden afternoon, that chimed in me with the sentiment of the song. It made me ache for home; but also made me think of life beyond the war, when things would all be good again – whenever that might come.

*

As if to deliberately break the rule, an epidemic did follow the earthquake in Haiti, and has since led to much confusion about the relationship of one to the other. However, examination of the circumstances confirms, rather than breaks, the rule. It was ten months after the earthquake had struck, before cholera was confirmed in Haiti, long after any direct effects of the earthquake and its unburied dead had gone, and for the first time there in more than a century. It was not the dead that were now threatening the living, but the threat lay in the living, condemned as they were to unsanitary conditions, with raw sewage flowing into rivers and streams, and sometimes down the streets. Cholera is transmitted by the faecal contamination of water and the accompanying lack of facilities to wash or to purify it before drinking. It was not endemic in Haiti, and so can only have been imported. Subsequent investigations, including identification of the particular strain, pointed to Nepalese peacekeepers as the source of the infection, although the UN has never formally taken responsibility. A tragic irony that hundreds of thousands of Haitians suffered, and thousands of them died, from a disease brought in by those sent there to help.

Having seen the surgical field hospital up and running, it was time to start the first rotation of our volunteers into and out of Haiti. I saw the first team off and welcomed the new team in. With only a few days left of my deployment I woke one morning feeling generally unwell. Not enough to worry me unduly and certainly not enough to stop me going into the hospital. On arrival there I began to feel weak and started to shiver. I rapidly got worse and remember asking for a chair, as I found I was simply unable to stand. Having sat down I said I had to lie down, and so became a patient in my own hospital. By now I was having rigors – a high temperature that leaves you feeling extremely cold – and shivering markedly. It looked like malaria.

Prior to coming to Haiti, I had been working in Uganda but had taken full malaria prophylaxis, which I continued to take while working in Haiti. However, the tablets are not always fully effective and subsequent testing showed that I had a serious case: falciparum malaria, the deadliest. So seriously ill was I that I had to be evacuated by air ambulance to Florida for further treatment. I was profoundly disappointed by what I considered to be some sort of failure on my part, but also extremely grateful for the care I received from my colleagues whilst in Haiti, and subsequently at the Mayo Clinic in Florida. It took me some weeks to recover, but I got back to work, and set about discussing with colleagues how we could once again look to improve the response to these large-scale events. The background to my vulnerability to malaria, in spite of taking the recommended prophylaxis, was eventually to become clearer, when a few years later I became very ill and was hospitalised once again, this time with whooping cough – an unusual illness in someone of my age. Subsequent investigations showed that my immune system had been compromised by my autoimmune disease and the heavy metal poisoning.

*

On returning to the UK I had an opportunity to read the press accounts of the disaster. I was particularly struck by the constant references to crowd violence and lawlessness in the population. Whilst there is a high background level of violence in Haiti, my personal experience was of a remarkably stoical people, acting more with than against each other. True, I did witness a temporary outburst of violence when a food parcel fell off the back of a truck and hungry people scuffled for its contents. But this was quickly over, and no one was seriously hurt that I could see. What lingers more in my memory was when driving out to Port-au-Prince to inspect field hospitals in the countryside, I saw a food distribution point where a few Haitian nationals were handing out sacks of rice to their compatriots who were queueing in a tight serpentine queue that twisted all the way round and across a large open square. The sacks of rice ready for distribution were piled openly beside the table where it was being distributed. Nobody broke out of the queue to simply pick one up and run away with it as they could have so easily done. Nobody complained. Everybody quietly waited their turn. There may have been an element of fear of summary justice from the crowd if anyone broke ranks, but I sensed something very much more. A display of community spirit you will not always find in similar circumstances, in other countries.

As devastating as the earthquake was, it did drive people together. Whilst doing a clinic in a small village in the hills, the residents were telling me how after the earthquake and the damage to the prison, the gangsters and criminals who had been terrorising their small community returned, and looked to take up from where they had left off. It was too much, a woman said to me. We had suffered enough and they were not going to take what little we had left – so, they hounded them all out and they didn't return.

Driving through the Haitian countryside revealed the absolute poverty in which so many live. Tumbledown shacks were home to whole families and more. Rivers of sewage ran through streets and alongside crumbled houses. Just how savage was the poverty became clear when I asked where the occupants of the post-earthquake houses in front of me had been taken. The answer was that the houses had been unaffected by the earthquake: they were like this before, and the occupants were still there.

Modern technology is beginning to improve the response to disasters and supported the response to the earthquake. As in many poor countries, mobile phones have a crucial part to play in communication, and in fact most aspects of everyday life and are ubiquitous in Haiti. Telecomms companies could track the exodus from Port-au-Prince after the earthquake by following mobile phone signals, and also warn the authorities and relief agencies of their pending return. In a sad irony, the mobile phone company's high-rise building in central Port-au-Prince was left undamaged by the earthquake. It was built to the standards only they could afford.

*

In the December of 2010, almost twelve months after the earthquake in Haiti, the World Health Organisation convened a meeting in Cuba to bring together experts in the field to address how best to improve the standards of foreign medical teams responding to disasters. I was invited to attend, as were representatives from MSF, the Red Cross and other well-established NGOs and relief organisations. It was a very fruitful meeting, the upshot of which was an agreement to establish a 'Foreign Medical Teams Working Group', chaired jointly by a representative of the NGO community, and WHO. I was elected as the NGO chair and our first task was to establish an agreed classification and minimum standards for foreign medical teams. The subsequent 'Blue Book' that followed allowed teams to know the standards they were expected to achieve, and countries receiving such teams to know more clearly what was on offer. This group matured into an established secretariat at WHO in Geneva, and WHO Emergency Medical Teams Initiative. Teams who wish to respond to disasters can now register with the WHO and be classified according to their capabilities.

The final piece in the jigsaw is to have their capabilities verified by WHO. The UK Emergency Medical Team, a consortium between UK Aid, the Fire and Rescue Service, Humanity and Inclusion, and UK-Med was the first European EMT to be verified. An Emergency Medical Teams Coordination Centre staffed by the host government and members of the WHO EMT initiative has also been developed and is established in the affected country very shortly after the appeal for international help has been made. Teams now register there on arrival, ready to be placed where they are most needed, and where checks can be made to ensure the capabilities of unverified teams are accurately reflected in their self-declared classification. When the next really big earthquake struck in Nepal in 2015 this system was fully implemented. There were no reported incidents of any inappropriate surgery, or indeed any malpractice by incoming medical teams. In fact, using the classification system, the Nepalese government, could identify three teams that did not in fact have the capabilities they had declared and were subsequently politely, but firmly, invited to leave the country.

Alongside these international developments, the British government carried out its own 'Humanitarian Emergency Response Review,' led by the late Lord Ashdown, and published in 2011. I was asked to give evidence to the review and emphasised the relative cost effectiveness of providing medical support in humanitarian emergencies. Government health economists reviewed data from the UK Fire and Rescue service, who had responded to the earthquake in Haiti, and data from the UK medical teams. They concluded that in terms of saving lives, medical teams were 'at least 100 times as cost effective' as the UK International Search and Rescue. That is not to say they have no place in the international response: that would be throwing the baby out with the bathwater. But the report recommended that in future the UK government would 'develop and deploy niche capabilities in a more focused way where they add value'; 'only use search and rescue in situations where the UK can genuinely add value'; and importantly for UK-Med, 'incorporate surgical teams into first phase deployments especially after earthquakes.' The report was well received by the UK government who accepted the recommendations. In discussing the report, the UK government at the time stated 'the UK will ensure that its humanitarian aid is delivered on the basis of need alone, and on the basis of humanity, impartiality, neutrality and independence (the humanitarian principles) in accordance with its key international commitments. We will maintain a principled, non-politicised approach to humanitarian aid.'

This commitment stands in sharp contrast with the current volte-face in British foreign policy where the Prime Minister has openly abandoned any such internationalism and has referred to aid as a 'cashpoint in the sky'. Appearing before a parliamentary committee he emphasised that he wanted to ensure that ODA (official development assistance) is better spent 'on serving the diplomatic, the political, the values of the UK, and indeed the commercial and employment (sic), the jobs interests of the UK.' This is the open expression of what I've witnessed in practice ever since I began working in international humanitarian assistance. As a legacy of empire, I'm sure, the FCO has seen overseas aid as a lever of power rather than an instrument to do good and relieve suffering. This was openly expressed by incorporating the aid programme into the FCO, embedded in the ODA. The ODA saw an expansion of its activities during the war in the Balkans, but its activities were always scrutinised by the FCO proper and sometimes undermined. In a bold and farsighted move, the incoming 1997 Labour government freed the ODA from its immediate political masters and set up the independent Department for International Development (DFID). It seemed to me the FCO never truly recognised DFID as independent of its political overseers, and constantly sought to influence, and sometimes undermine its activities. There are of course good reasons for those working overseas on behalf of the UK government to have the support and advice of the FCO, and DFID was often co-located with the FCO in its foreign embassies. Staff did move between the two. However, witnessing the relationship at close quarters, I felt, somewhat downheartedly, that it was only a matter of time before the FCO either wore down successive governments or found itself within a like-minded administration, and overseas aid be subsumed once again into the FCO. As much as it breaks my heart, that time has now come, and we find ourselves in the new age of the Foreign Commonwealth and Development Office.

Interestingly, in 2011, the government at the time only partially accepted the recommendation to 'work with NGOs to promote the concept of accreditation or certification.' As indicated earlier, there is a reluctance within the broader NGO community to be formally regulated, and a circumspection around professionalising the sector. I can see that as 'non-governmental' organisations NGOs wish to maintain their independence and not be regulated in their activities as regards to who, where, and when they should help. But a lack of regulation can also mean a lack of standards and a lack of full accountability. The caution in this aspect of the government's response to Paddy Ashdown's report, I fear, may reflect the lobbying that was done by large NGOs. If so, then it is not something I feel particularly proud of and reflects an underlying desire to maintain a freewheeling, buccaneering, swashbuckling approach to humanitarianism. Instead it stated it would 'actively support NGO leadership to solve the problems caused by huge numbers of them attending disasters.' So, some concession to the overwhelming evidence of too many, doing too much, with too little demonstrable benefit.

I have been supported in my work from the outset by key members of DFID from when they were in ODA. I raised with them the issue of the need for a national register of healthcare professionals willing to volunteer to deploy overseas and a supporting national training programme on my return from Armenia in 1988. Writing in the *British Medical Journal* in 1992, I said 'the Minister for Overseas Development has responded favourably to the repeated pleas of many for a register of the whereabouts and availability of experience medical staff.' It was to be another twenty years and several changes of minister until Justine Greening, Secretary of State for Overseas Development, announced to the press the activation of the UK International Emergency Trauma Register. It was very pleasing to read her statement describing the register as 'designed specifically to respond to situations where surgical expertise is required and will mean that the UK provides a timely and coordinated response to rapid onset disasters.' Although this had taken a long time to come to fruition, I knew that at one level, it had always been well received without anyone leaping the final hurdle that would transform it into policy. Jack Jones, a recently retired civil servant from DFID and a key player in the development of the UK's emergency humanitarian response, reassured me by saying words to the effect of, 'governments move in mysterious ways. If you submit an idea and it is not accepted, it may be for several reasons, including that it is not considered good enough or workable. But it might also be that for a variety of inter-locking political machinations, the time is not right. So, don't give up and keep resubmitting.'

I had already set up a small register of volunteers, and up until then was funding its administration myself. With official govern-ment support in place and the publicity that this generated, even more healthcare workers came forward to volunteer, and UK-Med now had the funds to train them. The consortium of MERLIN, HI and UK-Med we had established in Haiti came together more formally now as an official, government-funded, national team. Proof of concept was to be tested when a 'super typhoon' hit the Philippines in 2013. I deployed there with the new UK International Emergency Trauma Register team in what was to prove to be my final overseas emergency mission.

11.

See and Treat

Philippines

On 7 November 2013 the eye of the Super Typhoon Haiyan made its first landfall in the Philippines. Wind speeds were over 140 mph with gusts of almost 200 mph. Such was the scale of the devastation that it caused as it rampaged across the country, four days later, on 11 November, the Philippines Government appealed for international assistance. I was the medical leader of the team that flew to Manila on 13 November.

It was pleasing to note on our arrival in the Philippines just how much the changes we had sought to bring about following Haiti, particularly the establishment of the Foreign Medical Teams Working Group at WHO, had already been implemented. We had forwarded our medical and nursing registration details prior to departure to the Philippine Department of Health and so were formally authorised to practice in the Philippines from the moment of our arrival. There was a coordination centre for the reception of incoming medical teams, and the Ministry of Health was not only expecting our arrival but was already considering where the team might be best placed. Although the working group at WHO had only circulated for comment the 'Minimum Standards and

Classification for Foreign Medical Teams' a little over three months earlier, such was the need for a document of this type, it had been put to use immediately. I was surprised but immensely comforted to be asked on arrival how our team was to be 'classified' according to the new WHO standards.

On arrival we were interviewed by the Reuters News Agency on behalf of the international media, as well as by a group of local journalists. The principal line of questioning was around concerns being voiced about the national government response. We were cautious in our responses, as we wished to avoid being drawn into appearing to criticise our host government when we had only just arrived. Moreover, we had yet to see things for ourselves. So, we emphasised the complexity and severity of both the disaster and the geography, and that any country would struggle to cope in these circumstances. Attempts to recruit outsiders into criticism of the local government is common during all of these events, and something we've experienced since our very first foray into Armenia over thirty years ago. But the fact is that however well-prepared, however well resourced, there are simply some disasters of such magnitude that any government will struggle, particularly in the first few hours and days. The strength of the response is measured more accurately in how quickly order can be restored and systems put in place. So it's not that medical professionals avoid answering the question, in the manner of a politician. It's the opposite: we don't know the answer until we have experienced things for ourselves. In addition, we are always aware that any perceived criticism can be easily misinterpreted, amplified or misused.

I have been 'doorstepped' by journalists in the most unusual of places. Once in a hospital in China I turned a corner in a corridor to be confronted by a Chinese television crew. The gist of the questioning was 'why does China need help from foreigners? What is wrong with our system?' My answer, although it might sound contrived, was actually spontaneous and heartfelt. 'Nobody knows everything. Everybody knows something. Together we will know more.' I think it's original, although the sentiments are not. It was subsequently incorporated into a mural at Salford Royal Hospital when I was working there later. However, the most impressive response to 'doorstepping' I've witnessed was not mine. At the time the Right Hon Baroness Lynda Chalker was Minister for Overseas Development in ODA and was visiting to review the work being carried out in Sarajevo funded by the UK, including by me and my team. She was clearly trying to pack in as much as possible and was in a no-nonsense mood; although courteous and pleasant as always. I was trying to do the usual niceties, when she began to walk quickly into the hospital and said, and I paraphrase, 'cut the small talk and tell me in detail what you are spending the UK taxpayers money on.' I reeled out a long list of facts and figures as we moved at pace along the corridor, where seconds later, in response to a question by a BBC journalist on what the UK was doing to help the hospital, she gave an immediate, full and direct answer – spontaneously rattling out, without pausing or looking towards me, everything that I'd just told her. It was perhaps the most impressive piece of rapid assimilation and instant explanation of information I'd ever seen. The journalist certainly seemed happy.

The journalist's-eye view of disasters has to be matched, at least in some degree, to the practical possibilities of what can be achieved. For example, journalists will often hire helicopters, as they did in the Philippines, and fly over the disaster scene reporting the scale of devastation they see and lamenting the lack of relief effort: 'If we are here, why aren't they?' However, they can at times fail to appreciate, or at least report, that little can be delivered by helicopter. Anything of substance, and certainly anything sufficient to match the needs they are reporting, can often only be delivered by road. But roads are amongst the first casualties of disasters, either being destroyed by an earthquake, a landslide, a flood, or after a typhoon like this, blocked by falling trees. Only when the roads are cleared and repaired enough to accommodate heavily laden vehicles can aid of a substantial nature get through. In some circumstances, helicopters themselves become particularly scarce once a large-scale media response has been mounted, as the media have the cash to meet the rapidly escalating inflationary cost of these facilities, leaving rescue and relief workers with fewer options. I noted at the time too that 'journalists went out of their way to thank us and the people of the UK for their support and for sending the team.' It's a two-way thing. We all need to be aware of the demands placed upon each other and try our best to work together.

*

It was agreed with the local authorities that the team would be most effective if it were to travel on to the island of Cebu, lying some 100 miles south-east of the capital. We arrived in Cebu late in the evening but found there to be little information on the health needs outside of Cebu City. At first light the following day, armed with a small hand-held satellite phone, I set off with a local driver north-wards up the east coast of the island on a 'see and treat' mission. With me were Mr. Steve Mannion, an orthopaedic surgeon and longstanding colleague; Dr Andy Kent, an anaesthetist and veteran of Haiti and other disasters; and Rob Holden, then working with Save the Children International, and previously with DFID. We were to explore if there would be a need for the full team to be based at the northern tip of the island or if we should be split and perhaps work in support of other teams.

We travelled north to Bogo City, just over sixty miles north of Cebu City. At first everything appeared to be disturbingly normal, with roadside food stalls doing good business, and no apparent damage. But when we arrived just north of Sogod, about three quarters of the way there, the damage to buildings and infrastructure became gradually and then increasingly significant. At one point, you could see the path of the typhoon by standing in the road and looking northwards, where everything immediately in front was damaged: trees combed flat and all pointing in the same direction, houses collapsed and roofless, empty and desolate. Turning around 180 degrees on the same spot, everything you saw, right up to where you were standing, looked to be essentially normal. Trees and houses stood tall and straight, people strolled in the street, vendors sold fried chicken by the roadside.

Large-scale disasters, including typhoons, are a regular feature of life in the Philippines, and their emergency plans are well practised. I found them a remarkably resilient people. While children were asking for food and water at the roadside, they were also often playing and laughing, and thankfully, for the most part, did not look particularly ill or significantly distressed. There were no unburied dead and none of the locals expressed to us any concerns in this regard. It was clear there was already a burgeoning national relief programme in place, with food and water being distributed by municipal bodies, and telephone lines and infrastructure rapidly being repaired.

We visited the district hospital in Bogo city, a seventy-bed facility with maternity and basic surgical facilities on site. We were told it normally employs three local doctors and a small number of nurses. There we found the Israel Defense Forces (IDF) medical corps already encamped in the hospital grounds with, surprisingly to us, Philippines and IDF armed guards at the gates, and the Israeli flag flying over the main body of the hospital. The high level of security surprised us at first, as there was no evidence at all of any threat to us as we travelled the length of the route to the very tip of the island. We'd even stopped in towns on the way and got out of the vehicle to talk to local people. Everyone was very friendly and greeted us warmly, thanking us for our efforts. There was an obviously higher level of background poverty in the north of the island and the health care facilities were basic, but I never felt anything but safe. The IDF may however have felt unsafe for other reasons: the politics of the Middle East follow them wherever they deploy. In Haiti I remember many large international NGOs avoided collaboration with the IDF, either surreptitiously or at times overtly, lest they prejudice their missions in other countries, particularly Afghanistan. I know some members of the IDF medical corps very well, and they are sincere and highly motivated. But they are a military team, deploying in uniform, into a humanitarian setting. For some, whatever the reason for deployment, a military team cannot be regarded as a humanitarian team by definition. While they might adhere to the first principle of humanitarianism – relieving suffering wherever it is found – it is a struggle for many to accept that, as soldiers, they can be truly free to adhere to the other three agreed humanitarian principles of neutrality, impartiality and independence. Many international NGOs will not therefore, as a matter of principle, work with, or alongside military forces. But how truly independent any of us can truly be, when we are dependent on others for funding, is something we must each ask ourselves before, during, and after every deployment. Probably the only organisation in my experience that can claim to be truly fully independent is MSF France. They accept no government funding and raise all their money themselves from public donations, using it entirely independently according to what they find, and in strict adherence to all the humanitarian principles.

The role of the military in humanitarian responses and how NGOs might work with them was the focus of much attention recently when there was an urgent need to provide medical care to civilians very close to the frontline in Mosul. The Iraqi authorities would only allow civilian teams to deploy if they worked alongside their military forces. Many International NGOs, including MSF but also the ICRC, would not or could not go against their principles, and in spite of the obvious need, felt unable to respond. A paradox indeed. A humanitarian crisis to which many humanitarian organisations couldn't respond because of their humanitarian principles. WHO, as the 'agent of last resort', is obligated by international agreement to mount a response in such circumstances. They mobilised funding to pay three organisations to respond on their behalf, and in so doing, work alongside the Iraqi military forces. Those who eventually deployed were a private, for-profit, medical company, that recruited healthcare professionals at very high salaries; an evangelical Christian NGO; and a North American medical NGO. Perhaps not unsurprisingly the actions of WHO in deploying such a group of teams alongside military forces raised much comment, and indeed criticism, from within the humanitarian community. In response, WHO commissioned Johns Hopkins University in the US to investigate and provide an independent report. The researchers concluded, amongst other things, that 'WHO and its partners emphasised the humanitarian imperative to save lives above the other (humanitarian) principles such as independence and neutrality, and as some claimed impartiality.' They also added that 'medical teams working directly with a combatant force should not be identified as humanitarian groups.' A remarkable conclusion. So even if doing the right thing; it is not humanitarian because it doesn't conform to all the humanitarian principles.

The military and NGOs therefore make uncomfortable bedfellows, as they have ever since Florence Nightingale castigated the founder of the Red Cross, Henri Dunant, arguing that the Red Cross alleviated the responsibilities of warring governments. By providing aid on humanitarian grounds, she argued, on a voluntary basis and funded by charity, it would actually make it easier for armies to carry on killing one another. Would Florence Nightingale have similarly castigated WHO? What would she think of the military themselves carrying out humanitarian work outside of war? Members of the IDF medical corps have contributed their military experience to the development of the WHO Emergency Medical Teams programme, which from the outset, has always welcomed the inclusion of military teams and considered its minimum standards to be equally applicable to the military as to civilians when working in humanitarian emergencies. There are also other factors at play. The Israeli government sets great store by the imagery of the IDF carrying out 'humanitarian work' around the world, and are not alone in this regard. The Australian government goes so far as to promote the work of their medical assistance team in assisting their neighbours in the Pacific region under the banner of 'Deployment is Diplomacy.' There is likely to be an enlightened self-interest behind any government's deployment to humanitarian emergencies – some are just more open about it than others.

The IDF medical corps confirmed to us that they had been treating patients injured in the typhoon but added that they had largely been dealt with now, and they could deal with any other casualties that might present. They described treating mainly soft tissue injuries, mostly bruising, but were also treating penetrating injuries from flying nails and roof fragments as the tin rooves were ripped off by the force of the wind. At least one person had suffered a penetrating eye injury and subsequent blindness from these flying nails. As much as the Philippines prepares for typhoons, the lessons and experiences that have gone before cannot be drawn on effectively if there are not the financial resources to implement the lessons from other disasters. In the same Pacific region, Cyclone Tracey hit Darwin in the Northern Territories of Australia in 1974. It too wreaked havoc, and one of its features was also the deadly high-speed missiles of flying nails and roof fragments: lifted up and propelled by the high winds off the corrugated iron rooves of Darwin's buildings. Since then the law in Darwin has strictly enforced updated building regulations and prohibited rooves of this type. Although there have been further cyclones, this terrible pattern of injury has been avoided. It was therefore heart-breaking to see the same preventable injuries occurring with devastating consequences nearly forty years later. But the rich have the resources to move away from typhoon-vulnerable areas or the money to strengthen their houses. It's the poor that remain. Just as I'd seen the poor of Iran rebuilding their mudbrick homes into the side of the mountain from where they had just crumbled and fell, as they had done so many times before – they were simply too poor to choose otherwise.

Travelling north from Bogo, the damage was now extensive, with trees uprooted and debris strewn across the road. Again, we saw people asking for food and water along the roadside, but equally there was a very visible municipal food and water programme clearly already underway and a doctor in a small community clinic confirmed to us he had already received sufficient assistance.

When eventually meeting up again with the team back in Cebu, they reported that WHO and DoH were now most concerned about the remote small islands, out in the South China Sea. The typhoon had generated a devastating storm surge that had particularly affected the many remote islands off the northern tip of Cebu and the North West of Tacloban on the neighbouring larger island of Leyte. This was where the UK response was now to be directed.

Jon Barden, who had been deployed by DFID to support the coordination of the international response on the ground in the Philippines, proposed that the logistical barrier to us gaining access to these remote islands in the South China Sea might be crossed by hitching a ride on a Royal Navy warship, *HMS Daring*, currently on manoeuvres in the area. The ship and its crew were being tasked to distribute much needed material aid – water, food and shelter – as part of a military deployment called 'Operation Patwin'. Only a day after my musings on the IDF and whether military teams can be viewed as truly humanitarian, I found myself discussing 'embedding' my team with the British military for the purposes of delivering humanitarian assistance. There are established UN guidelines on the 'use of foreign military and civil defence assets in disaster relief', the so-called Oslo Guidelines, which I know British civil servants had first scrutinised in detail before suggesting we might join the warship. The Oslo Guidelines state that 'military and civil defence assets should be seen as a tool complementing existing relief mechanisms in order to provide specific support to specific requirements, in response to the acknowledged 'humanitarian gap' between the disaster needs that the relief community is being asked to satisfy and the resources available to meet them.' They go on to say that 'foreign military and civil defence assets should be requested only where there is no comparable civilian alternative and only the use of military or civil defence assets can meet a critical humanitarian need.'

It seemed clear to us that the only way we could get to, and around the remote islands in the South China Sea was by ship and helicopter. *HMS Daring* was in the area, had its own helicopter and small RIBs (rigid inflatable boats) to gain access to the islands, and could transport medical teams on and off. We were deploying alongside Save the Children International who I know had to discuss internally at the highest level as to whether they could/should deploy with the military. They too decided needs must. I and many of my close colleagues have always taken a somewhat pragmatic approach, and as long as the Philippine authorities and the UN coordinator were in agreement, which they were, we were happy to take advantage of the opportunity afforded to us by the Royal Navy. There were I understand discussions in the UK at Secretary of State level between the Ministries of Defence and International Development and ultimately the decision was passed up to Cabinet level. But in a very short period a cross government multiagency programme was put together and executed.

By early the following morning the medical team had the green light to go. Then, while making our final preparations for transfer to *HMS Daring*, we received a call from the head of the Australian Medical Assistance Team (AUSMAT), Dr Ian Norton, asking if he could draw from our numbers a surgical team to strengthen his in Tacloban. They were receiving a high number of patients who required emergency surgery, but it would take a further week for them to mobilise more surgeons from Australia. As we were already in country, they asked if we could bridge the gap. After urgent discussions between the Australian government's agency for the delivery of foreign aid (AusAID), DFID, UK-Med and Save the Children, it was agreed that six of the team, led by Mr Steve Mannion, would deploy immediately to the Australian field hospital in Tacloban, and the remainder deploy as planned with *HMS Daring*. I went with the bulk of the team to the port where we were met by the crew of *HMS Daring* who took us in a small motor launch towards my first foray onto a warship.

The launch pulled up alongside this huge ship, dangling down from the side of which was a slender, flexible ladder that had been rolled down from a hatch in the side of the ship, many feet above us. There was some anxiety amongst the team about how we would manage to climb up this and into the ship, and in a spirit of leadership, or perhaps of 'well I got you all into this', I said I would go first. To my surprise, and I expect the disappointment of all the onlookers, I negotiated the whole length of the side of the ship without falling off, and was duly welcomed aboard by Captain Angus Essenhigh. The captain was a remarkable man who seemed totally unfazed by a bunch of hippie humanitarians aboard his warship, and he helped our mission enormously. It came as no surprise to me that he went on to even bigger and better things, taking command of Britain's biggest warship, the aircraft carrier *HMS Queen Elizabeth*.

Along with the medical team, approximately one tonne of medical kit and supplies were loaded onto the ship. We were quickly introduced to the main ship's company and briefed on their mission: Operation Patwin. Aerial reconnaissance from the ship had identified several islands that had suffered significant damage and were clearly in need of assistance. Information from Manilla indicated the wider scale of devastation was beginning to be fully appreciated, with over 11 million people affected, over a third of whom had been displaced from their homes. Over 5,500 people were already known to have died and almost a further 18,000 were missing. At least 26,000 of the survivors had suffered injuries. Over 1 million homes had been damaged.

Fatalities were noted to be particularly high in Tacloban, where, as we had found in Cebu, a significant feature was injuries caused by flying debris, including penetrating wounds, lacerations, and contusions, compounded by infections caused by delayed or absent treatment. The decision to send the surgical component of our team to Tacloban seemed therefore to have been the right one.

*

Early the next morning, the day of my sixty-second birthday, I joined a four-person assessment team to the island of Guintacan. On giving my personal details to the flight controller as I was about to board the helicopter there appeared to be a problem. The upper age limit for flying in a military helicopter was apparently sixty years of age. 'But I'm here now,' I said. 'I suppose you are,' he replied, and on I got. We flew by helicopter from the ship, and as we flew over the island many of its 7,500 inhabitants ran out of their houses waving coloured towels to signal the aircraft to land, writing the word 'help' in the sand with their feet. They ran towards us as the helicopter landed on an open field and took us to meet with the local community leader, known on the islands as 'Captain'. She told us there were approximately 7,000 people on this small island that measured perhaps only 4 by 1.5 miles, grouped into three munici- pal areas or 'Barangays'. The island had six artesian wells from where water would normally be pumped into their houses, but they were now having to hand draw their water by buckets on ropes as there was no power. Not that it was that much better before the typhoon, but they did normally have power for about six hours a day. They were still able to pick up mobile phone signals so had contact with the outside world, although we were the first to deliver any assistance. She described how they knew the storm was coming but everyone chose to stay. Moving off the island was no small venture, and she described how there were people on the island who had never been off these 6 square miles of earth lying in the South China Sea. Instead, people had stayed in their houses, tending to move from smaller houses into neighbours' houses if they were bigger and stronger. In normal times a large supply boat kept the islanders stocked with essentials brought over from the neighbouring larger island, but this was lost in the storm. They had two boats remaining, but these were very much smaller which made getting adequate supplies onto the island problematic. There were no doctors on the island, but we were able to meet with a nurse and a midwife who provided healthcare to the whole of the island. I was also offered the use of the community leader's mobile phone to speak with the head of the Disaster Resilience and Response Council in Santa Fe, the main municipality on the neighbouring island, to ensure our work complemented the local and national assistance programmes.

I stayed on the island while the helicopter returned to the ship to begin ferrying in the full medical team. Once we were all ashore, we established a clinic at either end of the island, and working with the island's nurse and midwife, saw about 200 patients in the day. Most had been injured in the typhoon, but the islanders also took the opportunity of there being doctors on site and presented to us with long-standing, untreated conditions. These included a tumour of the parotid gland, a tumour in the breast, a basal cell carcinoma of the skin, thyroid problems, and tuberculosis. We worked with the island's health care staff to assess how best these patients might be referred onwards through their system, explaining the provisional diagnosis, and giving advice on how best to describe the condition.

Of particular concern to the islanders was the damage to the school roof and the destruction of at least one of the school buildings. The 'Captain' was very keen to receive our assistance in repairing the school and so allow the children to return. The children were restless and distressed she said, and she emphasised the importance of a return to a normal routine to help their psychological recovery. We found the 'captains' throughout the islands to be quite formidable people. The ones we met were women and commanded almost absolute authority. When I expressed a desire to inspect the health centre further up the island, the captain I was speaking with simply clicked her fingers at a passing youth on a motorcycle, who stopped immediately. After a short exchange of words, she summoned me to sit on the back of the machine and he promptly took me up and down and over a winding path to the north of the island. The child in me could not resist emailing home later from the ship that in one day I had been on a warship, a helicopter, and a motorcycle.

The Royal Navy distributed boxes of high energy biscuits and shelter kits to over 500 families. I watched in admiration as members of the ship's company set about repairing the school roof, cleaning its interior of debris, and cutting up and removing a huge tree that had been blown over and blocked its entrance. All done swiftly, efficiently and with huge good grace and humour, as we set about seeing patients. Injuries were mainly wounds and lacerations, but there were some more serious injuries including a wrist fracture that the team manipulated under local anaesthesia.

Over the following days the pattern was repeated across a series of small remote islands. Early start; helicopter and boat transfer of medical teams and Navy staff; work all day until nightfall; transfer back to the ship. The medical teams ran clinics while the naval staff repaired buildings, restored boat engines, and repaired generators. Some of the islanders spoke of a storm surge twenty feet in height. On one island, the artesian wells had been contaminated with sea water. Although the inhabitants were able to collect rainwater, this was in short supply. An islander therefore travelled to a neighbouring island each day to source 2,000 litres of fresh water. This lack of good quality drinking water led to dehydration in some of the children, who we treated with oral rehydration therapy and left ample supplies of these life-saving salts with the family. The Royal Navy provided adequate supplies of bottled water. We discovered more untreated fractures across the islands, including fractures to the hands and ankles. Fortunately, we could manage to reset these under local anaesthesia, and we had sufficient equipment to apply appropriate splintage. On every island we saw the now usual pattern of lacerations and other injuries from flying debris. The Royal Navy continued to distribute hundreds of boxes of high energy biscuits and thousands of litres of good quality drinking water. Each evening on return to the ship, we held a debrief with the senior naval officers and finalised our daily report. This was for both the UK government and importantly for the Philippine authorities and included the scale of damage to each of the islands we visited and an estimate of their projected needs in the coming weeks and months.

Meanwhile on Tacloban, the team found the extent of the

damage to be extremely severe – worse even than in the north of Cebu. Not only had many houses been flattened by the wind, but a storm surge many metres high had further devastated the low-lying areas of the City. They set about seeing up to 250 injured patients a day and began operating within forty-five minutes of their arrival. They were to ultimately carry out over 100 complex surgical procedures on those patients with more severe injuries. In five cases, sadly, the injuries to limbs were so extensive that limb salvage was not possible, and amputation was required. One of these patients was a small child whose injured leg had been left too long without treatment, and which was now so badly infected they had developed septicaemia and would have died without immediate amputation of the festering limb. Reconstructive surgery was possible for many patients, and included the surgical reconstruction of tendons and nerves, and the closure of open skull fractures.

Back on the islands, as we were about to leave Calagnaan, 200 miles north-west of Cebu City, and getting ready to return to the ship in good time before nightfall, a young islander pleaded with us to see his elderly grandmother who he said had suffered a serious injury to her hip area. We were worried from what he described that she might have a hip fracture, and so require a medical evacuation for surgery. Once we left the island, we would be sailing on overnight, and so this was her only chance for a while to get the treatment that would ease her pain and importantly get her mobile and so avoid all the complications that come with fractured hips in the elderly. We followed him to where she lay, much further away than we had understood or anticipated. It turned out that she hadn't fractured her hip, but rather had a large painful haematoma (collection of blood). We could reassure her family that it was safe to get her up and about, showed them how, and gave her a good supply of painkillers. But now darkness was beginning to fall and we needed to get back to the ship as soon as possible. The crew of the RIB had already been dispatched to bring us back to the ship when we asked them to wait while we set off to see our patient. They'd made it clear that they were under strict orders to be back on board before nightfall and had warned us that they would leave without us if it looked like we would not make it back in time. We just about managed to get to the rendezvous point before they left, wading waist high in the water to where the RIB already had its engines running, ready to race back to the ship.

A young naval rating hauled me unceremoniously over the side of the boat, and being last on, I took the seat at the front: the seat that would feel the most impact as this high-speed craft bounced up and down in the turbulent post-typhoon waters. The RIB took off at speed. The crew were clearly under pressure to return in time but there was also an element I thought of demonstrating to a bunch of civvies what it is really like to be in the Royal Navy. Whatever the reason, the boat sped through the still rough seas at increasing speed, with the crew giving no quarter to the inexperience of their civilian passengers, and the boat began lifting high up into the air over the waves and crashing down hard into what felt like a concrete slab of a sea. It was during one of these rough hard landings that I was thrown off the narrow bench seat and onto the floor of the boat. I managed to scramble back onto the bench, rather like an amateur horse rider scrambling over the back of a horse, head down, almost horizontal, clinging on for dear life. But by now I was completely unaware that the craft was high in the air and about to come crashing down even harder than it had done already. Before I was thrown from my seat I had been copying the more experienced in the boat and standing proud of the seat, like a horse rider standing in the stirrups over the saddle, taking the impacts of each landing in my legs while flexing my knees. Now, while remounting, as it were, with my head down and me yet to position my feet in the foot holes in the boat and get myself back into a brace position, I found myself sitting upright on the bench just at the moment the crash-down happened; and I was completely unprepared. I took the full force of the landing through my spine and felt an immediate and excruciating pain in the middle of my back. I knew I had broken it, I just didn't know how badly. I was in such pain I couldn't hold on and the naval rating behind me took hold of me and steadied me on the bench. Still the boat didn't slow down. The doctor who was seated near me later confessed she realised she had heard the bones break. Now began one of the hardest of times – the hardest I have ever had to bear.

As the boat approached the ship I began dreading having to climb up the side of the ship, but at least some luck was on my side, and this time we stayed in the boat while it was hauled up by a crane and onto the deck. I could barely move but forced myself to get up and out of the boat. I don't remember much of that evening. My colleagues realised I was in pain, but I was desperate not to disrupt the mission if it could be avoided, so I did my best to underplay my condition. I expected I may have slightly crushed the top of one of the vertebrae but told everyone I had badly pulled my back. My colleagues gave me strong painkillers and I went to my cabin earlier than usual. I was fortunate that I had the bottom bunk in a two-berth cabin. However, bunk beds on a warship have high sides to stop you falling out in a storm. For someone with vertebral fractures they seemed an almost insurmountable obstacle. I couldn't bend to get undressed so slowly and with increasing pain, I managed to get myself over the raised side of the cot and covered myself up top-to-

toe to avoid my cabin mate seeing me fully clothed and asking awkward questions. I was sharing my cabin with the Civilian–Military Liaison Officer from the Department for International Development, who had been stationed on board *HMS Daring* as part of Operation Patwin. If he were to see how injured I was he would no doubt feel obliged to tell the captain and we would run the risk of the medical component of the mission being aborted.

This was the first time a UK NGO had deployed with the military. I had long advocated for joint UK civilian–military deployments to humanitarian emergencies, given the massive logistical support the military can provide. The mission was already proving to be a complete vindication of this concept and I was determined to see it through, whatever the cost to me personally. You may consider this reckless. I thought it through as much as I could in the circumstances. I did not have any neurological symptoms or any other features that would require immediate surgery. I could station myself on board ship and so not put others at risk if they had to evacuate an island quickly. As long as I could tolerate the pain, I felt I should persevere.

That night the pain became simply unbearable. I realised there must have been swelling around the injury. I lay awake in agony and wondered in the morning how I could negotiate the high sides of the bunk bed. I mustn't let my roommate see me struggle so again I pretended to be asleep as he got dressed. When I heard the door close, I tried to sit up and realised even more just how serious were my injuries. Even lifting myself slightly provoked pain so great it was impossible to overcome, and I had to lie back, catch my breath, and wait for the pain to ease. To get up and out of bed over the cot sides seemed impossible. I would have to wait for someone to come looking for me then let events take their course. I tried and tried but just couldn't overcome the pain. But I kept trying and hoped the noise of the ship's engines would mask any screams of pain if I could really force myself. Closing my eyes and holding my breath I rolled sideways rather than attempting to sit up and, screaming in agony, rolled myself over the cot sides and fell onto the floor. The pain got even worse. I checked my legs and they were moving. I could feel everything, and I could hold onto my bladder and bowels. As far as I could tell, my spinal cord was still intact.

I slowly but surely pulled myself up by the side of the bed and into a half standing position. I negotiated the corridors and steps of the warship slowly and warily. Another fall and that really would be it. By the time I met up on deck with my colleagues I was pale and sweating, and they knew I was seriously injured. I was able to conceal the severity of my injury from the captain by dressing up my desire to stay on board in the guise of offering to be the on-board medical contact for the teams ashore on the islands; something he had already requested we organise. The team supplied me with regular strong painkilling medication, and I sat out the last week of the mission on board ship, as my colleagues carried out clinical work on the islands. On returning to the UK I realised there was in fact bleeding from the two fractures into the confined space of the surrounding soft tissues, which were coming under increasing pressure. I didn't quite realise it then, but this was to be my last mission to the field, and the start of my new career as a desk-based humanitarian: an armchair warrior.

The ship returned to Cebu to take on further stores and the medical team disembarked; but without me. I needed to hang on a bit to finalise arrangements for the incoming second team that would join *HMS Daring*'s sister ship, *HMS Illustrious*. The transfer to the shore was to be by the infamous RIB, so required a long climbdown from the ship that I simply couldn't manage. We agreed that I should stay on board to await a potential alternative. This materialised in the form of a Philippine launch that came alongside to deliver supplies to the ship, and after some negotiation with its crew, became my transport to the port. But the launch didn't stop where the big ships do, with gantries to the dockside, as I was expecting. Instead it drew up alongside the harbour wall, with its occupants expected to run up the twenty-foot high bank of car tyres that lined the harbour wall. Having borne so much, so far, my heart sank deep to the pit of my stomach. I couldn't fail now. I wouldn't fail now. As I scrambled up the tyres to the sailor on the dockside above me and his outstretched hand, I hoped above hope that the sailors on the launch would catch me if I fell. I found myself pulled sharply onto the dockside, panting, and almost fainting with pain, but knowing now that I was starting my journey home.

*

On my return to the UK, I rang a consultant orthopaedic surgeon friend of mine, and we met in his clinic shortly afterwards. X-rays showed one of my verterbrae crushed so badly that only a small disc-like fragment of bone remained; the other was crushed to about half its normal height. The worry now was for the spinal cord. I was transferred to the care of a neurosurgeon and had an MRI scan. When the scan was finished, the radiographer came into the room and lent over me as I lay on the scanner's table. 'Don't move' she said, 'lie perfectly flat and stay still'. She told me I was to be admitted immediately to the trauma ward. 'But I've been walking around for over a week' I said. And without irony or cruelty, but with brutal honesty, she leant over me, face-to-face, and said 'then more fool you'. She had a point. Not only were the vertebrae crushed, they had been fractured into several pieces, one of which had been pushed backwards towards the spinal cord itself. The lining membrane of the cord had been pushed inwards, but the bone fragment had not moved quite so far enough as to touch the spinal cord itself. I was a millimetre away from paralysis.

I was extremely well treated in Salford Royal Hospital, where I had been both a junior doctor thirty-five years earlier, and Hospital Dean a few years before. The multidisciplinary team came to the view that it was probably best now to let the fractures heal without surgical intervention, which could always be done later if I developed any major complications. After a week or so in hospital I was fitted with a surgical brace to keep my spine stable, and I was allowed home to convalesce. It took me three months to get mobile enough to consider going to work, but I did recover. Walking, standing or sitting for prolonged periods was very difficult, but I could manage with the aid of a stick, and by wearing the brace. I had lost height – probably 2 inches – and as the fibrosis around the fractures caused tightening of the tissues, the spine bent and twisted. I have been left with a permanent kyphoscoliosis: a forward and sideways curvature of the spine.

The fact that the fractures were so serious raised concerns that my bones may have been particularly thin. The chelation therapy that I'd received to treat the heavy metal poisoning had eventually begun to thin my bones and was one of the reasons why it had to be stopped. I had subsequently received excellent treatment for the thinning of the bones, and tests ultimately showed that normal bone density appeared to have been restored, but obviously not enough. The heavy metal poisoning from the Balkans was still taking its toll on me thirteen years later.

I had been fairly battered by all my work in emergencies and disasters, both physically and mentally. The cost had been enormous, and I was struggling to come to terms with my physical vulnerability. I also had to think long and hard about whether I had been reckless, and if my lack of concern for my own safety and welfare had put the safety and welfare of others at risk. It was time now to take stock.

12.

Flying a Desk

Gaza / Manchester / Sierra Leone

Ultimately, I was forced to retire from emergency medicine due to ill health. That decision has left a deep, unhealed wound. I have dreams to this day where I'm back at work in the Emergency Department, but something is always going wrong. Colleagues angrily ask me where I have been when I walk through the doors; I'm late for a shift and lost on streets I half know; I'm in the department and about to perform a life-saving procedure but can't remember how to do it. Sometimes each of these plays out on separate nights, sometimes altogether, but always with a sense of deep loss when I wake up. But at the time I still faced regular admission to hospital for one week a month for chelation therapy to remove the heavy metals from my system. But I was itching to make myself useful and I was determined to find a way of returning to some semblance of normal life. I spoke with my treating consultant and we agreed to move from intravenous therapy to oral doses. Although the treatment wasn't as powerful and would take longer, it didn't require my regular admission to hospital so I could return to working life.

I loved treating patients, and in particular combining clinical practice with an academic career. But retirement from frontline clinical medicine shifted the balance more towards the latter. I was appointed Emeritus Professor of Emergency Medicine at Keele University and I taught clinical anatomy at their new undergraduate medical school. I subsequently became Hospital Dean at one of the major teaching hospitals in Manchester, and I also began re-establishing my academic career at the University of Manchester, where I was subsequently appointed Professor of International Emergency Medicine.

It was there that I met Professors Bertrand Taithe and Tanja Müller. Bertrand's interests lay in the history of modern humanitarianism and I was keen to explore the background to humanitarian crises and those who respond to them. Over a coffee, Bertrand and I drafted a five-year plan for a new Institute, and put the proposal to the University. The day after my return from the earthquake in China there followed an impromptu and somewhat unstructured pitch to a potential benefactor, who very kindly offered us a significant start-up sum to establish the Institute straight away, rather than grow it over five years as we had proposed. A donation of this size would be matched pound for pound by the University, and so the University of Manchester's now world-leading Humanitarian and Conflict Response Institute (HCRI) was born. We recruited Dr Rony Brauman, former President of Médecins Sans Frontières (MSF) France to be the Director and I became its Deputy Director. It has gone from strength to strength since then, promoting research and teaching in humanitarian responses.

*

I have tried over the years to improve the approach to the management of emergencies at an institutional level, whether that be an emergency in a single patient, such as a sudden cardiac arrest;

several emergencies in the one patient, as occurs in those with multiple injuries; emergencies that affect many people, as in a major incident; or emergencies that effect hundreds of people, as in a major disaster. Each may seem very different from the other, but they have more in common than you might think, and for each we can prepare a plan.

I saw my work in international disasters as an extension of my work in emergency medicine at home. It's always important to question the rationale for the way things are done and to improve processes. The establishment of the Emergency Medical Teams initiative at the WHO after the earthquake in Haiti in 2010 was a leap forwards in the establishment of systems of medical care in large-scale disasters and humanitarian emergencies, and UK-Med played a key role in its development. The response to the typhoon in the Philippines in 2013 had shown the benefits of such a system in a sudden onset disaster, and nine months after my spinal injury, in 2014, I was asked by the UK government to test its use in war and mobilise a response to the conflict in Gaza. Working with our close colleagues, Humanity and Inclusion (then known as Handicap International), I despatched a surgical team, again led by Steve Mannion, and a follow-up rehabilitation team led by Peter Skelton. This was my first experience of leading from behind and I was not comfortable. Until then, no matter how dangerous the mission, I only ever asked team members to join me in a risk that I too shared. Now I was sending them into danger from the safety of my office. In darker moments, a taunting inner voice whispered to me of my cowardice. I had to tell myself repeatedly that this was how it was now; how it would always be. I simply had to accept my new position in the scheme of things, admire the bravery of others, and do my utmost to keep them safe.

As the casualties in Gaza mounted, the demands for international support for the injured grew, including pleas for their evacuation to safer places. Our surgical team was able to confirm what experience already predicted: all those severely injured from bombs and bullets would either have already been treated by the medical staff in Gaza or perished. The additional medical needs would be for the rehabilitation of the survivors. They found too that those in need of medical evacuation had found refuge in neighbouring, and Arabic-speaking, countries. The surgical part of the mission was therefore relatively short, but had provided an important first-hand, reliable, on the ground, assessment of the situation. The rehabilitation component, however, would last over six months.

Our work in Gaza raised our profile further across government departments, and particularly within the NHS, where senior figures recognised the value of both the register from which they could draw experts, and a national team of experts that they could deploy. Within a matter of months, this new relationship with the NHS led to a request to UK-Med to expand its role beyond mainly treating injuries and into the management of disease outbreak. The outbreak in question was the ebola epidemic in Sierra Leone.

*

Ebola virus disease, to give it its full title, was first identified in 1976 as one of a number of deadly viral haemorrhagic fevers. Haemorrhagic because they stop the blood clotting and those affected haemorrhage spontaneously and catastrophically. Prior to the epidemic in Sierra Leone there had been more than twenty outbreaks, primarily in remote rural villages in Central Africa near to tropical rainforests, with the largest historical outbreak occurring in 2000 and centred around Gulu, a small town in the north of Uganda. The nature of that outbreak had been recognised by the then medical supervisor of Gulu's St Mary's Hospital Lacur, Dr Mattew Lukwiya. Having identified both the nature of the infection and the scale of the threat it posed to the community, he alerted national and international authorities, and mobilised his hospital as an Ebola Treatment Centre (ETC). He worked tirelessly in the fight against ebola until he too became its victim. A great man, and a truly good doctor.

Ebola virus disease tells us a lot about our changing world. The virus is transmitted to us from wild animals, and fruit bats are considered to be the natural host. In the past it only infected people who lived in remote areas close to forests, and as it is such a rapidly fatal disease, people simply died before they could spread it beyond their small isolated communities. Yes, tragically small villages could be almost entirely wiped out, but it spread no further. But as ever-increasing numbers of people are moving into towns and cities, rapid urbanisation has now encroached upon once remote areas. Even though death can be just as rapid, survival can be just long enough to transmit the disease person-to-person in these very overcrowded, poor, and often unsanitary conditions. Some of the very poor have been forced into eating bush meat, and so have faced direct contamination from infected animals.

By August 2014 the World Health Organisation declared the ebola epidemic to be a 'public health emergency of international concern.' In response to the growing crisis, the UK Government committed its Armed Forces, NHS and public health workers to a programme of support to Sierra Leone. The original request to UK-Med from the UK Government was to recruit and train some eighty volunteers from the NHS to support Save the Children in the running of a treatment centre with twenty beds designed to care for infected health workers. However, the plans were quickly scaled up as the numbers of infected patients in Sierra Leone increased. Save The Children was joined by other NGOs, including International Medical Corps (IMC) from the United States, GOAL from the Republic of Ireland, EMERGENCY from Italy, and Médecins du Monde (MDM) from France; each of which established and managed treatment centres of between 80 and 100 beds across five districts in Sierra Leone. There followed a mass mobilisation of NHS volunteers, unprecedented in its scale, and even more remarkable in that its purpose was to help another country. Of course, there is always an element of enlightened self-interest in any act of apparent selflessness and altruism. It was clear the international community wanted to keep ebola confined to the countries in West Africa, and the UK certainly wanted to keep it away from our shores. But having been close to the effort at all levels, including Whitehall, I was moved by the overwhelming sense of altruism that drove the whole endeavour. UK-Med rapidly scaled up its NHS recruitment plan, and was supported greatly by a letter to all Chief Medical and Nursing Officers from the Chief Medical Officer for England, the Medical Director of NHS England, the Medical Director of Public Health England, and the Chief Nursing Officer for England, circulated to all NHS Medical Directors and Directors of Nursing. That letter provided guidance to NHS clinicians wishing to volunteer in support of the crisis, and directed them to UK-Med. The Chief Medical Officers for Scotland, Wales and Northern Ireland expressed similar support. The response from those in the NHS to these letters and the associated media coverage was immediate and humbling. We received 750 applications to UK-Med's newly formed UK International Emergency Medical Register for ebola within days, rising to over 2,000 by the time recruitment was closed. The awful dangers of exposure to ebola were by then very well-known, but nurses and doctors still came forward.

Volunteers were invited to an ebola information evening alternating each week between Manchester and London. As has been my practice from the start, it was emphasised that volunteers could withdraw with no questions asked and at any time. We were fortunate to benefit from the experience of nurse Will Pooley, who spoke to the meeting about his experiences of contracting ebola while working independently as a volunteer in Sierra Leone when the outbreak began. Following successful treatment at the Royal Free Hospital in London he was to return to Sierra Leone and resume his work. Other feats of heroism and bravery multiplied. One of the potential volunteers resigned his post in the NHS and volunteered to work independently in Sierra Leone rather than benefit from the special treatment afforded to NHS staff, who would be repatriated to the UK in the event that they became infected.

Of course, one of our members did contract ebola. Within a few hours of hearing the news, I received a call on my mobile from the Medical Director of the NHS, Sir Bruce Keogh. I expected him to say, not unreasonably, that the programme was to be halted. Not a bit of it. He asked me when the next ebola information evening was. 'I'll be there,' he said. True to his word, he turned up, as did every volunteer who had put their name down for the meeting; nobody withdrew. Sir Bruce gave a moving talk, explaining how growing up in Africa he had heard of this 'NHS' and marvelled at the altruism behind it and resolved to serve it when he grew up. Seeing one of our volunteers become so ill only strengthened his resolve, he said. It was one of the most moving and genuine speeches from such a senior official that I have heard.

We put all our volunteers through a health screening programme before they left and to avoid any perceived or actual conflict of interest, it was carried out by an independent health organisation. I didn't want any suggestion to be made that we would cut corners to recruit the number of volunteers we needed. Similarly, we offered no financial inducements to volunteers. The NHS would continue to pay their salary, but there was to be no extra 'danger money'. I wanted people to volunteer out of a desire to help and not be drawn by any financial reward, however much it might be deserved, or indeed needed. If the worst should happen, I wanted their sacrifice to have been for the noblest of motives. We did have to turn some away on grounds of health or other conditions. Four in particular precluded deployment. The first was pregnancy: immunological changes in pregnancy meant that pregnant women did badly if infected with ebola. The second was the presence of open skin lesions. These would obviously allow infected fluids to enter the body more easily, despite PPE. The third was if they refused to take malaria prophylaxis. This may sound odd, but there are healthcare workers who share the same anxieties as some in the general population around certain medications. There are also some who will simply not follow rules. When I was in Sierra Leone I discussed malaria prophylaxis with an aid worker who boasted they never took it. 'Aren't you afraid of getting malaria?' I asked. 'I've had it,' she said and proceeded to tell me how she had cerebral malaria, nearly died and required airlifting to Paris for treatment. Sierra Leone has one of the highest burdens of malaria in the world and the disease is one of its leading causes of death and illness. It also takes its deadliest form, falciparum, in over 85 per cent of cases. The final contraindication was the presence of any obvious significant psychological vulnerability. The stress of living under the constant fear of an almost certainly fatal infection, working all day in the heat and humidity of the tropics in full PPE, and witnessing so many people die in often horrific circumstances, is a huge psychological burden for anybody to bear. It would have been too much for those already suffering. In fact, it is well established that for those responding to traumatic events, a predictor of future psychological problems is the presence of pre-existing psychological vulnerability. Some of those who were rejected on health grounds took it badly. They had faced and overcome the obvious fears of what they were stepping up to and faced the anxiety and often anger of their family and friends. Some had even appeared in local newspapers and spoken on the local radio and been fêted as heroes. To be turned back now was at best disorientating for them and at worst a perceived humiliation, though I did my best to reassure them that the heroism was in the stepping up in the first place.

A complete mock-up of an Ebola Treatment Centre was built in York by the British Army, the air warmed to tropical levels to acclimatise the team to working in PPE in such stifling heat. Volunteers were taken through the treatment regimes and taught how to work safely, and, crucially, how to safely put on and remove their equipment. PPE is more familiar now in the era of Covid-19: face masks visors and gowns or aprons. But in Sierra Leone they had to wear full body PPE, with tight-fitting masks, double gloves, and large Wellington boots in 40°C and 80 per cent humidity. Volunteers described water 'pouring' from gloves and Wellington boots when 'doffing' their PPE, and losing around 3 litres of sweat in an hour. They went straight from the course venue by coach to the airport and onwards to their allocated ETCs in Sierra Leone.

The first group of NHS volunteers recruited through UK-Med deployed in November 2014 followed by a further seven teams, until requests for further international support reduced in April 2015. A further two teams were trained and held on standby until the programme closed in November 2015. Over 150 NHS volunteers were required to deploy and a further 40 were trained and held on standby. The programme could have deployed many more, but as more Sierra Leoneans were trained to work in the ETCs, and volunteers from other countries also came in support, the need for NHS support reduced.

Irrespective of ebola, it is estimated that over a third of those who deploy on a humanitarian mission report a deterioration in their health, either during or shortly after the deployment. The added threat to health care workers deploying into an ebola epidemic can only have increased these risks, and so we commissioned a post-deployment health screening of all the NHS volunteers. The commonest health complaint (40 per cent) was thankfully not too serious and perhaps not unsurprisingly the commonest health complaint of all travellers, particularly to the tropics: an upset stomach. We were of course looking out for signs of ebola as well as significant signs of psychological stress. The volunteers were also under separate surveillance by Public Health England (PHE) for the first twenty-one days of their return to the UK: the maximum incubation period of the ebola virus. Although never officially referred to as 'quarantine' to avoid worry, healthcare workers were 'restricted in their activities' during this period. This included having no patient contact, and as the virus is spread by contact with infected bodily fluids, no unprotected sex. Unlike Covid, you are not infectious with ebola until you get obvious symptoms; the viral load is simply too low until then. So, unless and until they had symptoms, our volunteers were in fact no risk to their patients. But such was the level of public alarm, including within the NHS itself, a blanket ban on patient contact was introduced. Then as now, there is always a balance to be struck between the hard scientific evidence and maintaining public confidence. Although the volunteers received their full salary during this three-week period, many were frustrated knowing that while they were symptom-free, they could be back with their colleagues doing their normal job. Some employers found them non patient-facing roles within the hospital during this period, but others simply asked them to stay away. For many this period proved the most challenging, and for a few an imposition too far. But it was imperative to maintain public confidence in what we were doing. They had signed up to the programme, which included the immediate post deployment period. Then as now, controlling the public message was difficult, and those in authority were not always in agreement. While our teams were overseas, a senior Public Health England official, was quoted in the *British Medical Journal* as saying that quarantining or restricting the movement of healthcare workers returning from countries affected by ebola virus disease was based on 'no science or bad science'. In the end everyone complied with the guidance, however they felt about it.

There was though understandable public terror at the thought of ebola, aggravated further by lurid accounts of the ghastly death suffered by those infected. But the risk was only to those in direct physical contact with the suffering. But as the virus is present in bodily fluids, and there in very high concentrations at the time of death, and for many hours afterwards, those who handle the dead are also at risk. The virus causes extensive bleeding and seepage of fluid, ultimately from every orifice, by the time of death, and inevitably contaminating the surface of the body. Burial practices where the relatives bathe the dead before internment, would expose those dressing the body to these highly infected fluids, which are then easily transferred from hand to mouth, or hand to eye, from where they are readily absorbed. This was a significant source of community spread in West Africa. The eventual introduction of safe burial practices was an important contributor to the control of infection, even though it meant families sacrificing many deep-rooted, and extremely important, cultural practices.

The hallmark of the onset of ebola and the start of the infectious period, is a rise in body temperature. Twenty-one of our volunteers developed a fever, either during their deployment or during their 21-day period of restricted activity on return to the UK. Although never reported in the press, thirteen of these volunteers were isolated in a hospital. Only one developed ebola. We had another volunteer who had travelled back on the same flight and developed a temperature on arrival home. She too was admitted to hospital for tests, all of which proved negative. All except for the ebola test, for which she was still awaiting the result when I spoke to her on the phone. I was still struggling with the responsibility of asking volunteers to follow me and take risks that I wouldn't share, and with these brave nurses now in hospital and potentially paying the ultimate price, I found it harder still to bear my sense of guilt. She immediately sensed the sadness and anxiety in my voice, swiftly turned the tables, calmly telling me not to worry. Here was someone who had risked everything, and may now be about to find out she had risked it all, in order to help others in a far-off country, and her only concern now was for me; the one who'd asked her to go. 'Whatever happens' she said, 'it was worth it'. She ultimately tested negative, made a good recovery and returned to her work as a Health Visitor as soon as she was out of hospital. When I later met her at an event where I'd spoken of her actions she said with genuine puzzlement that she didn't understand what I was making such a fuss about. I guess someone as selfless as her wouldn't.

*

Those close to me knew why I wasn't deploying, but I still felt profoundly guilty. In radio and television interviews I would sometimes be there alongside one or two of our young volunteers. The inevitable questions to me about whether I would also be deploying, and the look I thought I saw on the interviewers' faces when I said I wasn't, told me all that I needed to know about how I felt they viewed me: this armchair general, sending young people over the top and into battle. I never explained my position, rightly or wrongly, not wanting to become a story myself. So, I stuck it out. I certainly had more than enough work to do in the UK coordinating the response, but my internal pressure to deploy and share the risk eventually became too much and, unknown to my family, I referred myself for a pre-deployment medical. I failed. Because of my spinal fractures, I didn't have the physical ability to stand unaided for several hours in an ebola treatment centre and my residual immunological deficiency made me too vulnerable to the general threat of infection in Sierra Leone, let alone ebola.

Most volunteers thankfully suffered little lasting physical effects; remarkable given the physical hardships they had to endure. The psychological residue was also largely positive, reflecting a justified pride in what they had achieved. Sadly though, almost half of our volunteers described the social stigma they suffered on their return home. Many reported that friends refused to see them during the twenty-one-day post deployment period and a number were put under pressure by their employers to have no contact at all with their co-workers, even being asked not to return to their hospital accommodation. One doctor described being 'treated like a leper by many people' on his return and was uninvited from a wedding. A measure of the widespread, and rarely justified fear, was when after a visit to a bank to change back their Sierra Leonean Leones, a volunteer was telephoned at home by the bank manager who said an ambulance had been called to the branch as some of the staff were now experiencing 'symptoms'. Worse still, the police had been contacted, and the volunteer had to speak on the phone to the ambulance and police officers now in the bank, to reassure them no one in the bank was at risk.

Unsurprisingly, the volunteers themselves were riven with their own doubts and anxieties during this period of forced isolation. 'Ebola of the mind' they called it: a conviction that you've contracted ebola. This was particularly prevalent amongst those who returned when the press was full of stories of the one returning NHS volunteer who had been diagnosed with ebola. Some went so far as to describe these twenty-one days as the worst part of the whole trip: 'coming back to all the phone calls and the press and everyone's reaction to the news.'

The news they were referring to of course was that one of their colleagues had contracted ebola. I was at Heathrow Airport to greet that group of volunteers when they returned. One of the group told me after coming through immigration that she had concerns about the screening process. Everyone had been given a number for PHE, and we agreed she should call them. Eventually officials in yellow tabards arrived and took her back through immigration for further screening, and after about an hour they said that she was good to go. Shortly after she arrived home she became unwell, was admitted to hospital, and shortly afterwards diagnosed with ebola. Subsequently, a panel convened by her employers Save The

Children concluded that her infection was probably related to the use of PPE within their Ebola Treatment Centre.

She bore her illness and subsequent relapses with incredible fortitude. She suffered much exposure to press scrutiny and comment, some much less than kind, when in practice she had posed no real threat of infection to anyone else, even when travelling on the plane. Nevertheless, extensive contact tracing was carried out, more to alleviate public fears and in 'an abundance of caution', than to tackle any significant threat. PHE, then as now, also came in for criticism, but temperature screening at airports is a blunt and unreliable tool, and it failed in this case. As her condition worsened over Christmas, my worst fears were unfolding in front of me. But however I felt, it wasn't me that was lying close to death.

Her suffering didn't stop after her initial recovery. She was reported to her professional regulator, but subsequently cleared of any professional wrongdoing. I tried hard to find out who had done this to her, but no one would own up. The nearest I got from a senior official was that 'it came from the very top'. While altruism abounds in the NHS, a sense of fair play is not always as prevalent in its officials. On a later occasion, unrelated to this, I was summoned to meet with a senior Foreign Office official who demanded to know what I would say if 'a *Guardian* journalist was to ask me' about certain aspects of the government's mission in Sierra Leone. I reminded him that I was neither a civil servant nor a politician and would answer any such questions as accurately and honestly as I could. He jumped up from his chair, flung the door open, and said, and I quote, 'then f*ck off!'

On a happier note, in addition to a formal health screening programme, each volunteer had a telephone debrief with a UK-Med staff member, and with their permission we captured some of their comments. An independent review of these calls concluded 'there was an overriding sense that despite all obstacles, volunteers benefited hugely from the experience and felt they had achieved a great deal, which put many of the organisational challenges they met into perspective.' Volunteers were nevertheless deeply affected by the experience:

'You come back and you really start reflecting on things. The NHS has so much, gives you a different perspective on your own job, it will make me grateful.'

'First week back home was really difficult. I've got a two-year-old son and felt very sad when I saw him, just the discrepancy and the dichotomy in the world. Over a short period of time we saw a lot of people die. These thoughts have calmed down now, but I don't want to forget them. Talking with family has been hard, it's hard to explain what it's like to be in the Red Zone, it's so other worldly.'

'It was the saddest and happiest experience of my life'.

Recruiting staff from the NHS was not without its critics, but this was a global health emergency affecting a country with an already severely strained health service. Without outside support the epidemic would have continued for longer; the death toll risen even higher, and the long-term effects on an already impoverished country's population, economy and health service been even greater. To mitigate any risk to the NHS, volunteers were never drawn from any service known to be under pressure, and only one volunteer was drawn from any one department at any one time. The overriding principles were that the UK NHS service provision and patient safety would never be compromised; and there is no evidence that I have seen that it was.

In the end, it must be appreciated that it was Sierra Leonean healthcare workers who ultimately fought and won the battle against ebola, though the NHS programme was an important kick starter for wider international support for their efforts. The legacy for the NHS was a cadre of healthcare workers highly experienced in managing so called 'High Consequence Infectious Diseases', who were better prepared, and could prepare others, to respond both nationally and internationally when the next outbreak of a dangerous pathogen occurred. An initial rush of enthusiasm followed, and I was invited to sit on a High Consequence Infectious Diseases committee of the NHS and PHE. We started work on establishing a common training pathway for overseas and national deployments to reinforce our capacity here in the UK, but interest faded and eventually disappeared. Worse still, rather than pay for the relatively small cost of its storage, an official told me they were instructed to burn the remaining very large and expensive stock of PPE. Five years later the inevitable happened and the outbreak we could have prepared for so much better, fell upon us while we were sleeping.

13.

Humanitarianism Begins At Home

In my experience, the reasons people do humanitarian work are multiple: religion; a simple desire to do good; politics; and, yes, vanity, fame, and even fortune, can all play a part. What has made it worth it for me are not the first and the last of these, but the second: a simple desire to do good. But to achieve it, I've been drawn into the world of politics, flattered myself into vanity, and although never famous, have flirted with the media. But what makes it humanitarian? What does this word really mean?

When we hear the word 'humanitarian' nowadays, we usually assume that it implies an inherent goodness. But there have been too many instances of well-documented abuse associated with humanitarian organisations for this to be a given. Humanitarian work has also become glamourised by celebrity, and for me, correspondingly trivialised at times. Joining the 'humanitarian club' requires no special entry qualification, just the confidence to declare oneself a member. But it was not always so. Humanitarianism has meant so much more than this, and was recognisable in some of the most profound social movements taking place in the nineteenth century: movements that included the abolition of the slave trade and the foundation of the International Committee of the Red Cross (ICRC) in Geneva. At the heart of humanitarianism then, as it should be now, was a willingness to do things that are obviously to the advantage of others, but offer little advantage to yourself and might even be to your obvious disadvantage. That is, altruism.

When, during the American Civil War, Abraham Lincoln sought to cripple the economy of the South by blockading its ports and preventing the export of the cotton it produced, it was not only the southern states that were brought to their knees. The cotton now rotting on the quaysides had been destined to feed the cotton mills of Lancashire, including my hometown of Manchester, or 'Cottonopolis' as it was known, which in turn fed the people who worked in them. No cotton meant no food, and so followed the four years of the Lancashire Cotton Famine, from 1861 to 1865. But with the suffering came a remarkable act of altruism by the millworkers, who wrote 'in the name of the working people of Manchester' to Abraham Lincoln in support of the Union in its fight against slavery proclaiming 'The vast progress which you have made in the short space of twenty months fills us with hope that every stain on your freedom will shortly be removed, and that the erasure of that foul blot on civilisation and Christianity – chattel slavery – during your presidency, will cause the name of Abraham Lincoln to be honoured and revered by posterity.' In other words, their own suffering was worth it. Abraham Lincoln himself wrote back to the mill workers saying 'under these circumstances I cannot but regard your decisive utterances upon the question as an instance of sublime Christian heroism which has not been surpassed in any age or country.' The letter still resides in Manchester Town Hall today, near to the statue of Abraham Lincoln in Manchester's

Lincoln Square. But not only did the Lancashire Cotton Famine mark an early act of humanitarianism by the millworkers, it also marked the advent of mass fundraising for emergency humanitarian assistance. The Lancashire and Cheshire Operatives Relief Fund was set up in 1862, and donations rolled in from not only the United Kingdom, but from across its empire, and ultimately from around the world. Over £45 million in today's money was raised to feed the hungry, and the food itself was distributed according to need; a need identified by the daily calorific requirements that had only recently been scientifically established, and that we still basically use today.

These shifts in the social tectonic plates drew on the concepts of compassion, individuality, and most importantly reform. They were not just responding to terrible wrongs, suffering and injustice, but they were looking to also enact changes that would ensure they could not happen again. This element of reform is what is too often missing from modern day humanitarianism. If we don't dig down to the root causes of why people end up in such desperate need and remove them, this endless cycle of crisis, response and crisis will only continue. There are more than 10 million NGOs worldwide and such is the scale of the aid industry that it has been estimated if they all operated as one, they would be the fifth largest economy in the world. Bringing these vast resources to bear in a more concerted way would yield results. And when the root of the need for humanitarian assistance lies in the vulnerability brought about by poverty, then we need the same reforming spirit that abolished the slave trade mobilised to abolish poverty.

Whether we like to admit it or not, vanity and other forms of self-interest will often, and for many of us always, be a part of 'doing good': whether to win your place in heaven, to seek the approval and even adulation of others, or simply to feel good about yourself. It is hopefully not the only reason, and in my experience, for most people, it is not the dominant one. But in responding to emergencies and disasters there is also an element of adventure, and some more than others are drawn to risk-taking. I recognise this in myself. When speaking to potential volunteers I have asked them to be honest with themselves about these aspects of their motivation, and reassured them that such feelings do not cancel out, and probably do not even compare with, their overriding desire to step up and help.

But good intentions alone are not enough. They should be the starting point, not the endpoint. That must surely be when something has changed for the better. The desire to do good, to lead a worthy life, and to 'flourish' are ancient, and were established within both Western and Eastern philosophies long before Islam, Christianity and other religious commandments. They predate Aristotle, who described such desires as 'eudaimonia' and explored the concept of virtue: the desire to do good simply for its own sake.[14] And beyond religion's 'Divine Command' to do good, they evolved through the Age of Enlightenment to a fundamental duty – Kant's 'categorical imperative' – to do what's right, simply for its own sake and as an end in itself. All these values drive people to respond to help people they see as in need and in distress. The goodness is perceived as lying solely in the doing. But Aristotle warned us that being virtuous requires not only that you do good, but that you do it in the right way, to the right degree, and for the right reason. And 2,000 years later the philosopher Jeremy Bentham added the missing piece in this moral jigsaw, and demanded we also examine the goodness or otherwise of what we have done.

*

I have seen as much good work and as many good people in hospitals in the UK as I have doing humanitarian work overseas. Perhaps more. I have never forgotten as a little boy proudly telling my mother as we sat on the back seat together while travelling home on the bus that 'when I grow up I'll go on the Missions and help the people in Africa.' 'Oh, that's nice,' she said. 'But if it's helping people you're after you don't have to wait until you're older, and you certainly don't need to go all the way to Africa. You can start now. The old woman up the road needs help and I certainly do.' I took her point and remember it daily. In later life a senior nurse taught me again about the value of taking the opportunities around you to do some good. Simply and without fanfare. This operating theatre nurse told me about a senior orthopaedic surgeon who had a reputation for a degree of grumpiness and a short temper, although I personally found that his willingness to come to my assistance in the Emergency Department at any time, day or night, far outweighed any possible issues with his demeanour. One morning she went into the surgeons' coffee room and told the group of consultant surgeons there that a nurse had her purse stolen that morning and to be careful with their belongings. Many mutterings of sympathy and many platitudes followed, but it was only the late Mr Peter Frank FRCS who followed the nurse back to her office and asked how much was in the purse, before handing over the full amount in cash. Peter Frank had been in a concentration camp as a child, trekked across Europe to his freedom, and still bore his tattooed number on his arm. No wonder he didn't suffer fools gladly. And he'd learned that it was what you did that mattered, far more than what you said.

Since I began working in emergencies of one kind or another over forty years ago, I have seen enormous changes, most of which have been for the better. From the 'Casualty' departments of the 1960s through the 'Accident and Emergency Departments' of the 1970s and 80s, to the 'Emergency Departments' of today, the care of the acutely ill and injured has been transformed and established now as a specialty in its own right. None of this came easily but was achieved by the dedication of the nurses and doctors who have worked tirelessly over the years, and under the most difficult conditions, to step up and give of themselves when we have needed them most. When I started out as a medical student, the ambulance service wasn't even part of the NHS – now it is its backbone. The response by emergency medical teams to disasters overseas has now been put on a much more professional footing, with the establishment of a dedicated initiative at WHO in Geneva that has established international core standards and a classification system that allows countries to know exactly what they are getting and identify what they don't need. Lessons were learned from the mistakes of Haiti and those mistakes have never been repeated.

When I first responded as a doctor to large-scale humanitarian emergencies it seemed at times as though the rules that govern medical practice at home did not apply: these patients were different. I and other colleagues have fought hard to remind us all that patients are the same wherever they are and deserve the same from their doctors whoever they are. The UK now has a government-funded national emergency medical team, drawing from a pool of enormous expertise and providing a fully trained specialist response wherever, and whenever, it is needed.

UK-Med, the charity that I founded and now chair, recruits and trains the healthcare professionals for the national team, which also includes the UK International Search and Rescue Team and our long-term colleagues in Humanity and Inclusion. This combines emergency medical care, search and rescue, and rehabilitation in the one team that was the first in Europe to gain formal verification of its standards by WHO. UK-Med also deploys independently, funded by the money it raises. It has over 2,000 volunteers on its registers and has teams working all around the world. Hand in hand with its emergency response efforts it works with local health care professionals to increase their own capacity to respond. In 2014, UK-Med responded to requests for assistance to Syria by running training courses across the region in the complex management of injured patients exposed to the chemical weapons that were used. After responding to the ebola outbreak in West Africa we have deployed teams to the diphtheria outbreak in the Rohingya population in Bangladesh and subsequently to a measles outbreak in Samoa. At the time of writing the team has successfully completed a mission in Beirut following the terrible explosion there. UK-Med has sent teams to over 20 countries to support their Covid-19 responses, spanning Africa, Asia, and this Pacific, with a team having just left for the Solomon Islands.

*

Do I think it was all worth it? Yes, I do.

There is an immeasurable benefit in humanitarian work and the hand of friendship has a profound effect on those who receive it. I'm often asked though how I cope with having seen so much death, destruction, misery and cruelty. Surely it must leave me wretched and sad, people say. It would be almost facetious of me to say it has not affected me. I cope because that's only part of what I've seen. The overwhelming legacy, the abiding memory, is of the goodness that I've watched rise above and outshine all the rest. My thoughts are much more of how human beings know altruism, and seen in the aftermath of war the greatest act of altruism is that of forgiveness. My mind is filled with thoughts of the kindness and generosity shown to me by those who have had so very little and lost what little they had. The spirit of hope and perseverance shown by people in the very darkest of hours. I have learned that life is fragile and must be lived to the full. I've learned that human grief can know no bounds so we must treasure those around us now. People never get over a great loss, but with time and the support of others they may just learn to live with it: so let's help each other.

I've seen that the veneer of civilisation is thin and it cracks with remarkable ease. We have to be vigilant. But I've seen too that there are more resilient people than there are vulnerable, so the strong must help the weak. And in the end, there are no natural disasters: one way or another, they are all man made. It is the poor that always suffer as a result and the very poor that suffer the most. As poverty is the product of economics and politics, so it can be changed. We can do that, if we really want to.

I travelled in and out of Sarajevo over thirty times in under four years. Many times I felt the wall of air hitting me before I heard the explosion of the grenade; heard the whistle of a sniper bullet inches above my head; lost friends and colleagues, and more than one by their own hand. As my work there was drawing to a close for the last time, I drew together a meeting of the senior staff in the city's main hospital in order to reflect upon, and learn from, all the work we'd done together over those difficult years. At the end I asked the group to tell me what was the most important thing we'd done. Without hesitation they replied:

'You came.'

Postscript
Siren Song

In her poem, *Siren Song*, Margaret Atwood takes the ancient legends of sirens and mermaids – those lustrous female creatures who lured sailors to their beauty, only for them to be dashed on the rocks where they lay – and imagines they sang not merely of their beauty, but also of their vulnerability. They sang to the sailors, she says, of how they were helpless and in distress, and it was only they that could save them.

The sailors left the safety of their ships to swim to the rescue of those they could never save and died drowning in the sea of their supposed altruism and vanity. Accusations of 'vanity', 'attention seeking' and 'virtue signalling', are not new. All have been levelled at me at one time or another. But if people are being helped, do the motives behind their actions really matter? Does vanity diminish its benefits? Does doing good require you to be good? I have found the hungry hand to take before it questions, so the responsibility must rest with the giver – with me.

If there has been a driving force behind my work, it is that what you do matters at least as much as what you mean to do – and for me it matters more. I have heard that siren call and leapt overboard to swim to those in distress; towards those who, deep down, I may have believed only I could save. In undertaking humanitarian missions around the world, I have taken enormous risks with my life and with the welfare of those I love, and who love me. If the worst had happened, as it nearly did too many times, could I have said, like the nurse waiting for the results of her ebola test, 'it was worth it'? Could they? For me the worth lies in what was achieved, although the achievements in humanitarian crises are not always tangible.

Humanitarian action, as we know it today, and certainly in the West, has evolved largely out of the experiences of Henri Dunant, the founder of the Red Cross, and his observations of the aftermath of the Battle of Solferino. What he saw was the total and shameful neglect of those wounded in battle. He put it all down on paper in his book *A Memory of Solferino*. In the book he wrote 'what an attraction it would be for noble and compassionate hearts, and for chivalrous spirits, to confront the same dangers as the warrior of their own free will, in a spirit of peace, for the purpose of comfort from the motive of self-sacrifice,' and so invoked a raft of virtues to mobilise like-minded spirits. Or, as Margaret Atwood put it more bluntly, 'to leap overboard in squadrons.'

Not everyone heard the siren call. Remember Florence Nightingale's, letter to Henri Dunant saying that an organisation like the Red Cross would make it easier for armies to carry on killing one another? Just as my work in Sarajevo may have done. Just as 'Live Aid' was criticised later. David Rieff, writing in the *Guardian* in 2005, charged Bob Geldof's efforts for Ethiopia with helping to fund 'a brutal resettlement programme that may have killed up to 100,000.'[15] Not directly, but as Nightingale might have said, by relieving the burden from the perpetrators. Rieff claimed that 'as many lives may have been lost due to the indirect consequences of the aid as were saved by its direct benefit.' He quoted Bob Geldof, the architect of Live Aid, saying in response to such criticism, that 'we've got to give aid without worrying about population transfers.' And therein lies the rub. I'm a great admirer of both Band Aid and Live Aid, but Rieff did put his finger on the desire to do without looking at all the consequences of what you've done. He asked, 'Isn't it better to do something rather than give in to cynicism and do nothing?' I agree. Cynicism produces nothing and looks to justify doing nothing. But doing nothing is never neutral. I agree something must be done, but I also make myself look at what it is best to do, and what will do the most good and avoid harm. Rieff answered his own question about doing *something* by saying 'of course, those who believe it is always better to do something tend to believe that any negative consequences of their action arise from not doing enough.' I would go further and say negative consequences arise not from a failure to do enough, but our failure to do the right thing, in the right way, and for the right reasons.

If the world had stood by and not intervened in Sarajevo, then no doubt the Serbs would have rapidly taken the city. No doubt many civilians would have died, maybe many hundreds, but perhaps fewer than a thousand. But the world did intervene, and the war then lasted almost four years, with at least five times as many civilians, and many more combatants, losing their lives. If lives saved were the only measure of whether it was worth it, then it was not. But is this the right or only measure? I saw in Sarajevo, people who were prepared to die to protect the things and values they lived for, both in the recipients and the givers of the humanitarian aid. Florence Nightingale's approach, however logical, lacked humanity. Doing nothing, I tell myself repeatedly, is never neutral. Ignoring the suffering before you, to prevent suffering that may occur later, is something that is very damaging to the human spirit.

We now call it moral injury: 'the psychological distress which results from actions, or the lack of them, which violate someone's moral or ethical code.' We know, for example, that UK International Search and Rescue Teams rarely save any lives responding to earthquakes overseas. From what I can gather, the most they've ever saved was three, and that was in Haiti. They usually save no one. But when they are asked for help by countries in distress, should they say it's not worth it? I have stood in front of crushed buildings alongside the relatives of those trapped deep within while international rescue teams give them one last throw of the dice. Even though this is rarely, if ever, successful, it may provide the comfort of knowing that at least everything possible had been done. The very act of responding has value. The very act of refusing to respond has consequences. What might be dismissed as a gesture, can also be seen as an act of solidarity: of showing people they are not suffering alone in the dark. And that is why I responded to Sarajevo. I was asked, and having seen their agony, I couldn't abandon them.

Henri Dunant was also undeterred by Florence Nightingale, and quickly established the International Committee of the Red Cross (ICRC) in Geneva, followed shortly afterwards by the first of what were to be several 'Geneva Conventions'. The work of the ICRC has shaped humanitarianism ever since, seeing the development of International Humanitarian Law and leading to the first three humanitarian principles of humanity, neutrality, and impartiality being adopted and endorsed by the UN General Assembly in 1991. In 2004, Independence was added as the fourth core principle that underpins humanitarian action. It is a commitment to an adherence to these four humanitarian principles – humanity, neutrality, impartiality, and independence – that now defines an individual or an organisation as truly humanitarian.

The first principle – humanity – dictates that human suffering must be addressed wherever it is found. In so doing we must remain neutral in hostilities and refrain from engaging in controversies of a political, racial, religious or ideological nature. What we do must be impartial and carried out on the basis of need alone, giving priority to the most urgent cases of distress and making no distinctions on the basis of nationality, race, gender, religion, class or political opinions. Finally, we must be independent of any political, economic, military, or other objectives when humanitarian action is implemented. It is the first of these principles, however, that in practice is always the prime driver and sits most comfortably with all our motivations. In combination they form at times an almost unstoppable force, but if the driver is to act without any thought for the consequences, then real harm can be done, either knowingly or unknowingly.

We have come a long way since the earthquake in Armenia, with our good intentions but also mistakes. Much of my work since then has been to make sure we never make those mistakes again and furthermore that our desire to do good is matched by an equal capacity to do it well. To match altruism with professionalism. The former is never in short supply amongst healthcare workers, particularly those working in the NHS, but the latter has needed careful explanation and development. It requires underlining to those willing to volunteer that their altruism is the starting point and not the end, and that the professionalism they show in their everyday work through special training, qualification, and accountability, must be extended to humanitarian emergencies. Developing training programmes and a professional home for humanitarian healthcare workers has been essential. UK-Med provides core training, and WHO has defined core standards, for emergency medical teams. The final piece of the jigsaw for me was put in place in 2020 when the Royal College of Surgeons of Edinburgh established the Faculty of Remote Rural and Humanitarian Healthcare to give humanitarian healthcare workers the same professional recognition and support they have given any other healthcare practice.

However much I may look back still and wish that I had done things better, I gain some reassurance that I have at least been part of a movement that recognised its shortcomings and looked to put things right. Humanitarian work is still not perfect, but nothing ever is – and it is more needed now than ever before.

UK-Med has continued to respond wherever conflict is to be found. We have maintained an office in Myanmar in spite of all the difficulties and established an office in Yemen which was until recently the site of the world's largest humanitarian crisis. The conflict in Ukraine has overtaken Yemen in the race to hell. But there too UK-Med has teams on the front line, providing essential emergency healthcare and emergency surgery to the wounded.

I salute the bravery of the Ukrainians who resist and those who bear the pain of separation. Scenes of cities besieged and civilians trapped beneath merciless shelling bring back painful memories. The suffering endured by a mother who loses a child is always the same, wherever it may be.

Acknowledgements

I have written everything exactly as I believe I saw it at the time, and certainly as I remember it now. If others remember it differently, then so be it. This is my honest reflection on all that has transpired through what for me has been a turbulent lifetime of work. I did not though do these things alone. I have been frugal with name-checks in the text in order to smooth the narrative and to avoid disappointing those I would inevitably fail to mention. But there are some I must pay special attention to and document my heartfelt thanks.

Firstly, my wife Caroline and my daughters Katy, Sarah and Helen, who have hopefully forgiven me now for all the stress I have caused them. Very sadly my eldest brother Brian died shortly before publication but lives on in our hearts and memories. A special mention too for my grandchildren, Thea, Oliver and Rosa, whose names I promised would appear in my book.

When I came up with the concept of SMART it was enthusiastically supported by three friends and colleagues. The late, and very great, Dr J. Denis Edwards was one of the most gifted physicians I have ever had the privilege to work with and shaped much of the way I approached the care of the critically ill. Dr Brendan Ryan was my Registrar at the time and gave me unflinching loyalty and support, travelling with me to Armenia Iran and Kurdistan. He went on to become a Medical Director of great distinction. Dr Stewart Watson was already an established plastic hand and reconstructive surgeon at the time, and joined us on many difficult and dangerous missions, bringing with him his considerable surgical expertise for the benefit of the most vulnerable of people. He also garnered the support of the British Association of Plastic Reconstructive and Aesthetic surgery (BAPRAS) that formed the bedrock of 'Operation Phoenix' in Sarajevo. In addition to these three clinical colleagues, Philip Suker and Lynn May were original trustees of SMART and later trustees of UK-Med and have shown continuing support for the work, giving freely of their time over many years.

Establishing UK-Med would not have been possible without the unwavering support of Dr Mark Prescott. We became colleagues as consultants at the North Staffordshire Trauma Centre where he both gave me the space to be released from my work within the NHS when I travelled alone and worked alongside me on many a mission. He is the emergency physician I aspired to be and someone I am truly proud to call my friend.

Space does not allow me to name everyone who joined the various deployments but I would wish to pay special thanks to everyone who volunteered for 'Operation Irma' and 'Operation Phoenix'. In Sarajevo, nurses, allied health professionals and doctors from across the United Kingdom joined us in what was inevitably a very dangerous environment. They all came forward willingly and I'm truly grateful for their support.

When I thought illness had put paid to my exploits overseas, I was approached by Dr Amjid Mohammed, a consultant emergency physician, and Dr Waseem Saeed, a consultant plastic and reconstructive surgeon. Following their own work in the Kashmir earthquake they were looking to improve and expand what they could do, and rather than set up their own NGO, they threw their lot in with UK-Med and stimulated and galvanized a resurgence of our work.

All the teams who responded from the NHS to the outbreak of Ebola in Sierra Leone have my unqualified admiration. But they could not have got there without the untiring dedication of the team back in the UK, led by Roy Daly. Roy jumped ship across the university to support my work in global health and I have never forgotten his show of faith in me and what I was trying to do.

Professor Tanja Muller at the University of Manchester played matchmaker between Professor Bertrand Taithe, Professor of Cultural History, and myself, leading to the establishment of the Humanitarian and Conflict Response Institute at the University of Manchester: a unique marriage between the faculties of humanities and medicine.

From the very beginning of my international work I have worked closely with first the Overseas Development Administration and then the Department for International Development. My key contact in both these organisations and for all the time I was involved in this frontline work was Jack Jones. The words civil servant or government official do not do him justice. He was far more than that. He was extremely able and dedicated, but most importantly, a true humanitarian. I owe him a great deal and welcome this opportunity to thank him publicly.

A key player in the Department for International Development during the ebola crisis was Jon Barden. He worked tirelessly and effectively and subsequently played a pivotal role in UK-Med securing the funding to establish my life's ambition of a national register of healthcare professionals willing to volunteer to be trained for deployment to sudden onset disasters overseas. He became a good friend and we still work together through our work at WHO.

Finally, I want to acknowledge the new generation who have picked up the baton and are now running with it faster and further than I ever could, especially my colleagues at UK-Med – ably led by David Wightwick – and the Humanitarian and Conflict Response Institute.

If there has been a theme to my work, it has been to 'normalise' the medical care of the most vulnerable. 'Normal' medical practice is informed by evidence and supported by training, guided by established professional and educational bodies. The World Health Organisation, under the then leadership of Margaret Chan, established the Emergency Medical Teams initiative with its publication of essential core standards for foreign medical teams and Professor Michael Lavelle-Jones, when President of the Royal College of Surgeons of Edinburgh, personally supported the establishment of a Faculty of Remote Rural and Humanitarian Healthcare within the college and Professor Michael Griffin who saw it through to fruition. These two developments for me personally represent the culmination of the efforts I and so many others have made for so long to bring humanitarian healthcare firmly into the fold of good medical practice. I am truly grateful to these and other medical leaders, who used their power and influence to such good effect.

Acronyms and Abbreviations

APC – Armoured personnel carrier

AUSMAT – Australian Medical Assistance Team

DEC – Disasters Emergency Committee

DFID – Department for International Development, UK Government

EMT – Emergency Medical Teams

ETC – Ebola Treatment Centre

FCO – Foreign and Commonwealth Office, UK Government

HCRI – Humanitarian and Conflict Response Institute, University of Manchester

ICRC – International Committee of the Red Cross

IDF – Israel Defense Forces

INSARAG – International Search and Rescue Advisory Group

IOM – International Organisation for Migration

IRA – Irish Republican Army

ISAR – International Search and Rescue

IV – Intravenous

KLA – Kosovo Liberation Army

MDM – Médecins du monde

MEDEVAC – Medical Evacuation

MERLIN – Medical Emergency Relief International

MSF – Médecins Sans Frontières, Doctors Without Borders

NHS – National Health Service

ODA – Overseas Development Agency, UK Government

PAHO – Pan American Health Organization

PHE – Public Health England

Acronyms and Abbreviations

PLA – People's Liberation Army

PPE – Personal Protective Equipment

RIB – Rigid inflatable boat

RUF – Revolutionary United Front, Sierra Leone

SMART – South Manchester Accident Rescue Team

UN – United Nations

UNAMSIL – United Nations Mission in Sierra Leone

UNDAC – United Nations Disaster and Assessment Coordination Team

UNICEF – United Nations Children's Fund

UNMIK – United Nations Mission in Kosovo

UNPROFOR – United Nations Protection Force

WHO – The World Health Organisation

Notes

1. https://www.theguardian.com/world/2020/apr/14/england-coronavirus-testing-has-not-risen-fast-enough-science-chief
2. Humanitarian aid is material and logistic assistance to people who need help. It is usually short-term help until the long-term help by the government and other institutions replaces it. Among the people in need are the homeless, refugees, and victims of natural disasters, wars, and famines.
3. A not-for-profit international development company
4. Deontology is the normative ethical theory that the morality of an action should be based on whether that action itself is right or wrong under a series of rules, rather than based on the consequences of the action.
5. Utilitarianism is a family of normative ethical theories that prescribe actions that maximize happiness and well-being for all affected individuals. Consequentialism is a theory that suggests an action is good or bad depending on its outcome. An action that brings about more benefit than harm is good, while an action that causes more harm than benefit is not.
6. Humanitarian principles are a set of guidelines that govern the way humanitarian action is carried out. They are considered essential to establishing and maintaining access to affected populations in natural disasters or complex emergency situations. Compliance with the principles is an essential element of humanitarian coordination. The main humanitarian principles have been adopted by the United Nations General Assembly, and include: Humanity, Neutrality, Impartiality and Independence.
7. After Mary B. Anderson's *Do No Harm: How Aid Can Support Peace*, Lynne Rienner Publishers, 1999.

8. Opisthotonos is a spasm of the muscles causing backward arching of the head, neck, and spine, as in severe tetanus, some kinds of meningitis, and strychnine poisoning.

9. Kurdistan Workers' Party, a Kurdish militant political organization and armed guerrilla movement, which has historically operated throughout Greater Kurdistan, but is now primarily based in the mountainous Kurdish-majority regions of southeastern Turkey and northern Iraq.

10. Claus Von Stauffenberg was a German army officer best known for his failed attempt on 20 July 1944 to assassinate Adolf Hitler at the Wolf's Lair and remove the Nazi Party from power.

11. The Italian authorities would not accept the bodies without a death certificate. But there were no official death certificates yet for Kosovo, which although under UN administration was still part of Serbia. There was a definite impasse that seemed for a while to be unsolvable. I broke the deadlock by going to meet with the UNMIK regional Administrator and simply saying that if Kosovo were independent ('it's not,' he kept saying) but if it was. 'I would in effect be the Chief Medical officer and you the Head of Local Government.' In such circumstances we could issue a death certificate. I feel I wore him down until he didn't say no. So I made up and printed off the 'Medical certificates of death' and faxed them across to Rome. I did wonder if I had overstepped the mark and repercussions might follow, but none came. In retrospect I expect everyone was grateful to just get these poor souls home.

12. Josef Mengele, the 'Angel of Death', SS officer and physician during World War II remembered for his actions at Auschwitz; and Albert Schweitzer, winner of the 1952 Nobel Peace Prize for his philosophy of 'Reverence for Life'

13. The Revolutionary United Front (RUF) was a rebel army that fought a failed eleven-year war in Sierra Leone, starting in 1991 and ending in 2002. It later developed into a political party, which still exists today.

14. In Aristotelian ethics, eudaimonia is the condition of human flourishing or of living well.

15. David Rieff, 'Cruel to be kind', *The Guardian*, 24 June 2005, https://www. theguardian.com/world/2005/jun/24/g8.debtrelief

Index

Index

Index

Harper
North

Book Credits

HarperNorth would like to thank the following staff and contributors for their involvement in making this book a reality:

Hannah Avery	Megan Jones
Fionnuala Barrett	Jean-Marie Kelly
Claire Boal	Dan Mogford
Charlotte Brown	Simon Moore
Sarah Burke	Ben Murphy
Alan Cracknell	Alice Murphy-Pyle
Aya Daghem	Adam Murray
Jonathan de Peyer	Melissa Okusanya
Anna Derkacz	Genevieve Pegg
Gavin Dunn	Agnes Rigou
Tom Dunstan	Dean Russell
Kate Elton	James Ryan
Mick Fawcett	Florence Shepherd
Nick Fawcett	Zoe Shine
Simon Gerratt	Eleanor Slater
Alice Gomer	Hannah Stamp
Monica Green	Emma Sullivan
Lauren Harris	Katrina Troy
Tara Hiatt	Phillipa Walker
Graham Holmes	

For more unmissable reads,
sign up to the HarperNorth newsletter at
www.harpernorth.co.uk

or find us on Twitter at
@HarperNorthUK

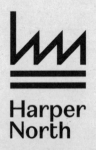

**Harper
North**